Your Demise Will Arise

Don't Close Your Eyes

by: r. pasinski de

•

Your Demise Will Arise

Don't Close Your Eyes

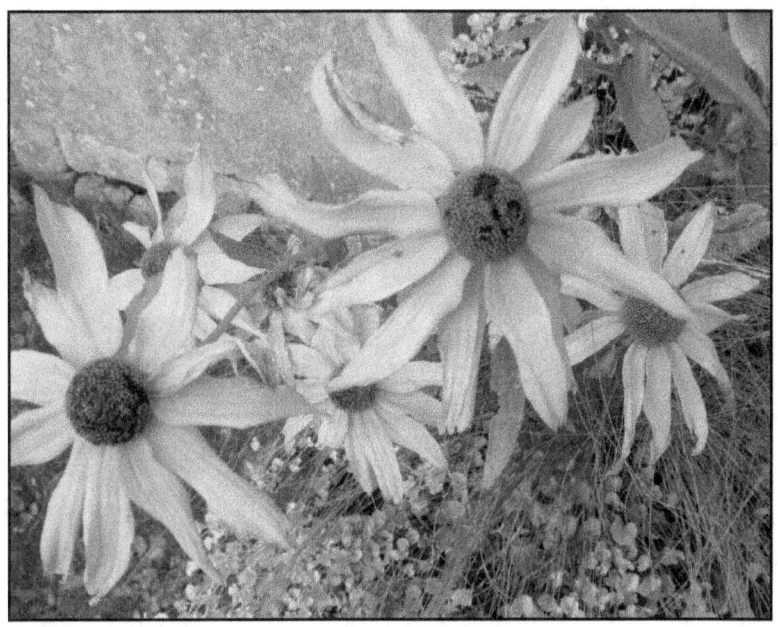

PREFACE

Your Demise Will Arise; Don't Close Your Eyes an insightful guide filled with numerous mnemonics. Reminders to keep our eyes open thereby attain a well-balanced, harmonious life by accepting the fact of life that you and I and everyone we know needs s to realize, that their demise, as well as our death, will arise one day. These short but to the point reminders can help us bring to mind the fact that our death will occur, and one day death will find all of us, so we need not close our eyes to that fact, to that Fact of Life.

For greatest retention, these mnemonics work best when taken on a limited and regular basis. One or two reminders a week works best for most people. Try to keep them in mind throughout the day but don't stress out.

This handy, pocket-size guide gives you easy access to contemplate existence and start being comfortable with thereby accepting the impermanence of life.

Remembering that one-day death will arise so don't close your eyes; you have no choice; not accepting your eventual demise is not an option. Death, yours and others, is a Fact of Life and if ignored may lead to a fragmented life.

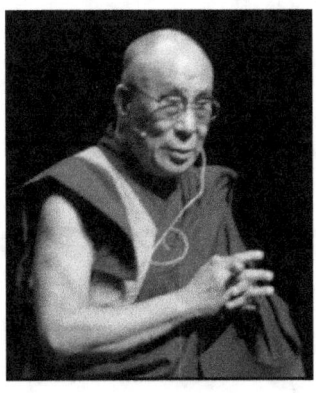

"Death is a part of all our lives. Whether we like it or not, it is bound to happen. Instead of avoiding thinking about it, it is better to understand its meaning. We all have the same body, the same human flesh, and therefore we will all die. There is a big difference, of course, between natural death and accidental death, but basically death will come sooner or later. If from the beginning your attitude is 'Yes, death is part of our lives,' then it may be easier to face."

Dalai Lama 1935-

•

•

•

•

•

•

•

•

Your

Demise

Will

Arise

Don't Close
Your Eyes

•

•

•

•

•

•

•

•

•

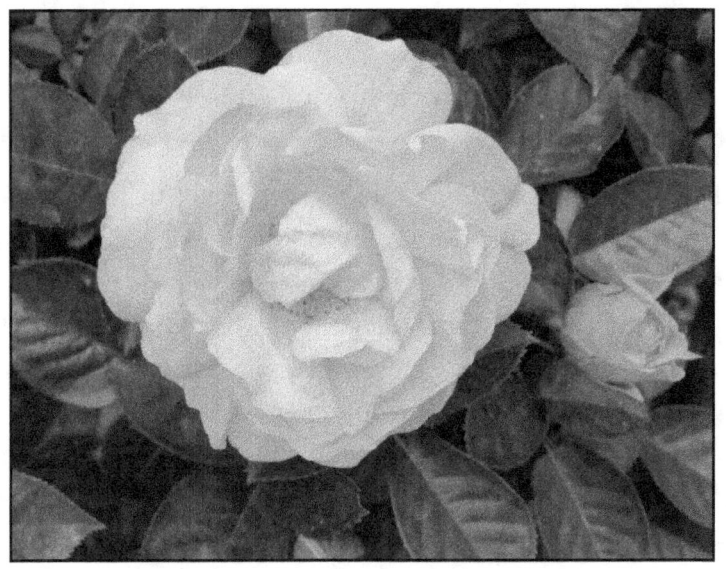

THE PROBLEM

The Problem Started

When We Were Born.

Our Folks Never Stated:

One Day They

One Day We

Would Not Be.

•

THE PROBLEM

The problem started when we were born. Our folks never stated, one day they, one day we, would be gone. Most parents never tell their children what death is, what it does, they never informed them that one-day death would come by and close their eyes, that one day everyone's else's demise would also arise.

Why didn't they talk to us when we were young about death? Probably because they feared death themselves, fear based on not realizing, not understanding that death comes with life, life comes with death. Life and death are conjoined twins; you can't have one without the other. They can't be separated. We have a choice to either see death as a problem or as a fact of life. When we see it as a problem, we're wasting time because it is a problem that will never be solved. The only way to look at death is to accept it as a fact of life, the fact that it will end our life one day. There is no escaping it. We have no choice but to open our eyes to our soon to arrive (could happen at any time) demise.

•

•

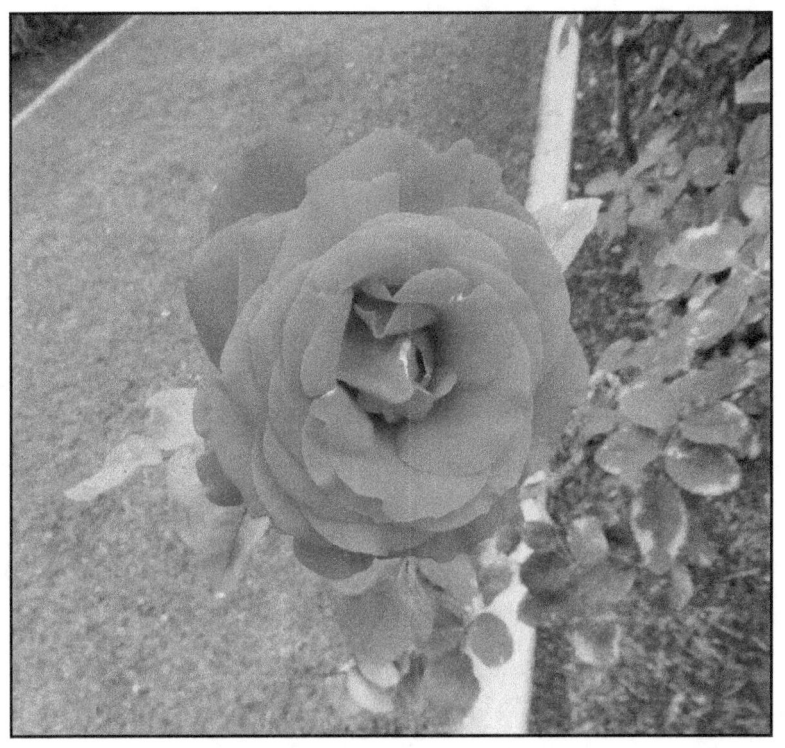

AN EMPTY SHELL

One Day We're Here

Next Day We're Gone

What's Left Is an Empty Shell

From An Era, Long Gone

•

AN EMPTY SHELL

One day we're here, next day we're gone; what's left is an empty shell from an era, long gone.

We are all empty shells when we're born. As time passes, we start learning how to control our shell aka body and start filling it, covering it, protecting it with life's tangibles and intangibles. And when our demise arises, our body will release everything that we clung to it over the years, and be an empty shell again like the empty clam and oyster shells we find on the beach, when we are laid to rest.

•

•

•

•

•

•

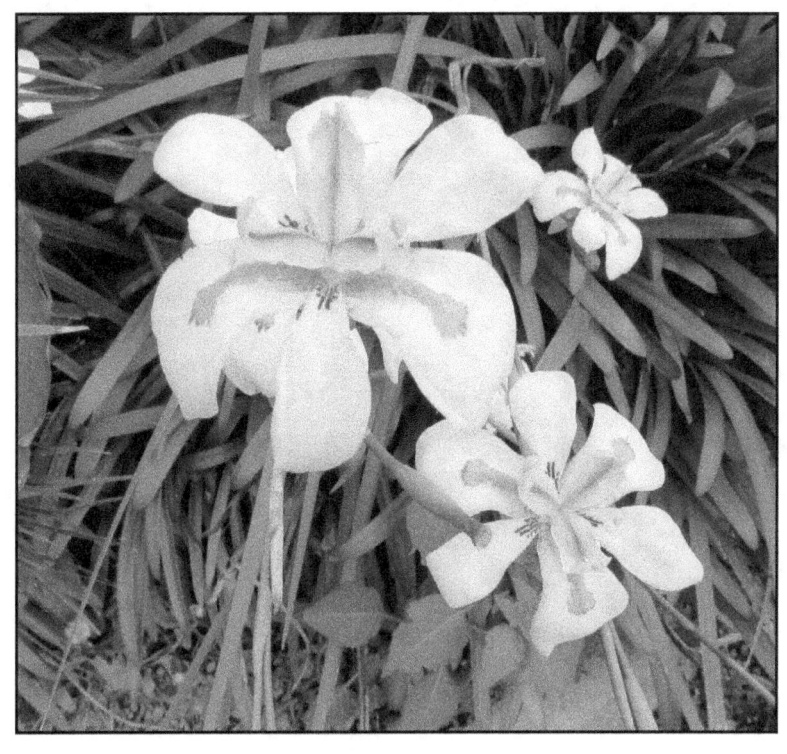

EVERYTHING

One Day We'll Be Buried

If One Day We're Not Burned

Leaving All Our Mates

And Everything

We Owned of Late

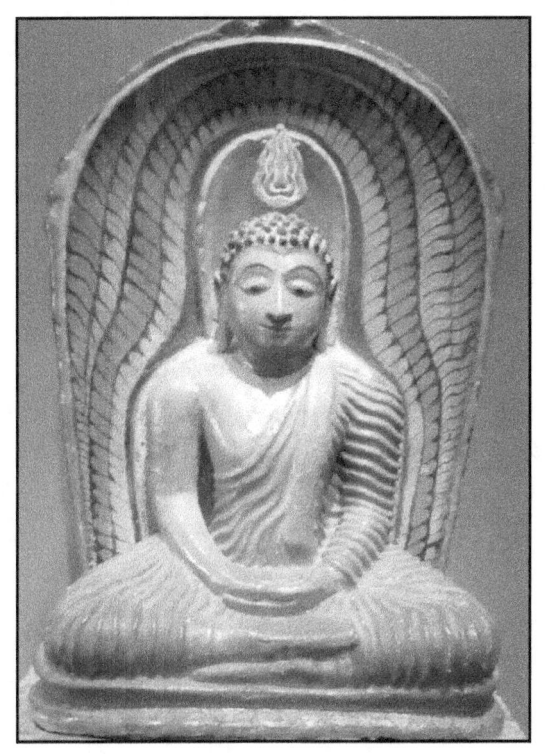

OUR SPOT

One Day We're Animated

Next Day We're Not

What Happened?

Death Found Our Spot

•

●

OUR SPOT

One Day We're Animated; Next Day We're Not. What Happened? Death Found Our Spot. One day we'll be going along singing our daily song, enjoying the sun or shade, the rain or snow and our demise will arise. Death will come by and says Hi, and start singing its song and tell us it's time to move on, time to say goodbye; our life has come to its end, our time has come to die.

●

●

●

●

●

●

●

●

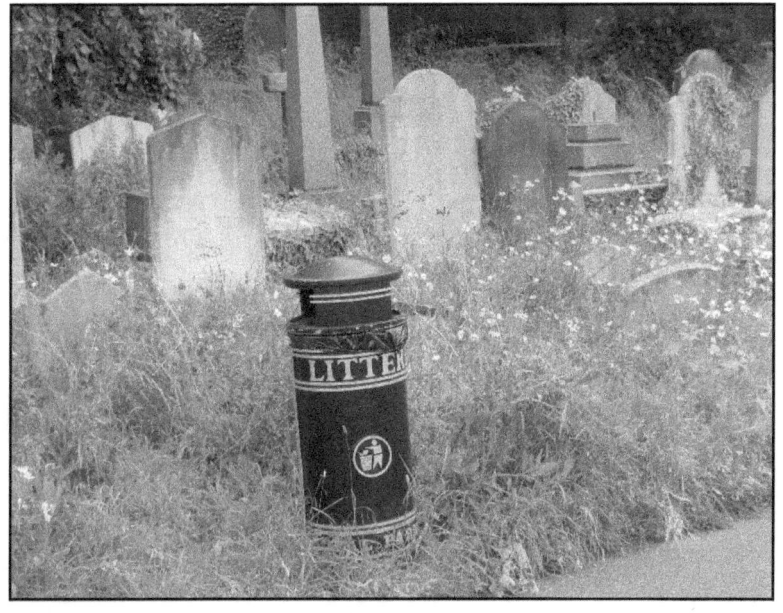

MONEY

Why Argue About Money?

After We Die

We Won't Need Any; Honey

•

MONEY

Why argue about money? After we die we won't need any; honey. Your money will not be needed when your demise arises. You won't need your purse in your hearse. All of your cash will stay back for your friends and family to enjoy until their death occurs, it's their time to follow your footsteps to the grave.

•

•

•

•

•

•

•

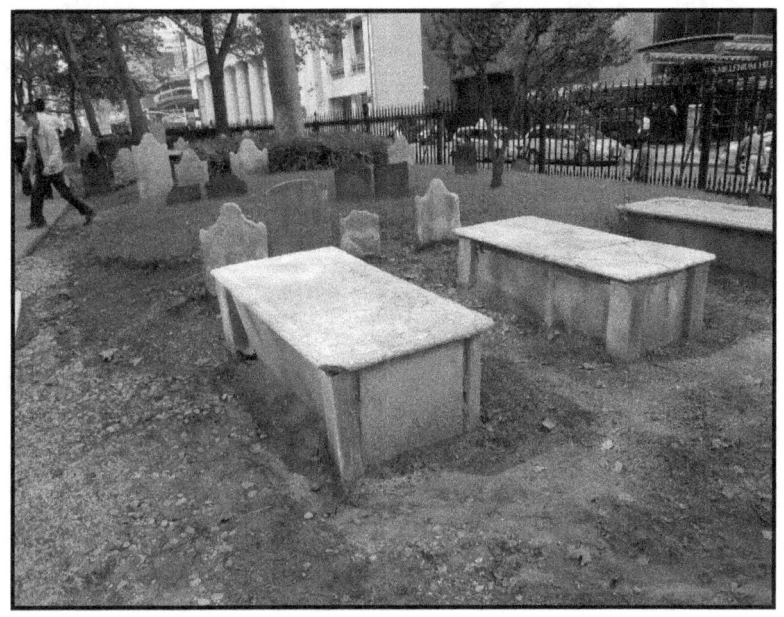

THE COFFIN

From the Perspective

of a Coffin

Life Looks Really Good

•

THE COFFIN

From the perspective of a coffin: life looks magnificent. At a Wake aka funeral would you rather be the guy or gal on the inside or the outside of the box? Most of us would choose the latter.

We need to start taking advantage of that freedom and start enjoying the outside before it's our turn to be on the inside, of the box, inside the coffin. A shiny new coffin surrounded by sweet smelling flowers, notes on condolences and a long line of tearful mourners, some sad, some indifferent, while others, some internally jubilant, waiting for the circus to end, waiting to collect their bounty.

•

•

•

•

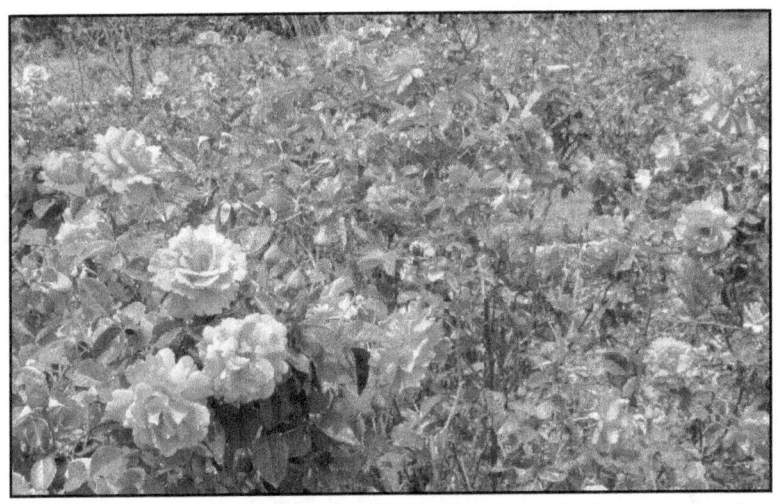

DON'T WORRY

Today Could Be

The Last Day of Your Life.

Don't Worry Be Happy

Why! Waste Time

Being Anything Else

•

DON'T WORRY

Today may be the last day of your life. Don't worry be happy. Why waste time, being anything else? Everyone's death is at hand hiding somewhere in their future; realize it! It's catching up with all of us, getting closer and closer with each passing day and will be here sooner than we think.

One day we'll step out of this timeline and our time in this world will have ended, and we will again be nonexistent.

So let's not waste this time, this day, today and seize the time we have now, it may be gone tomorrow. Seize it before it's too late.

•

•

•

•

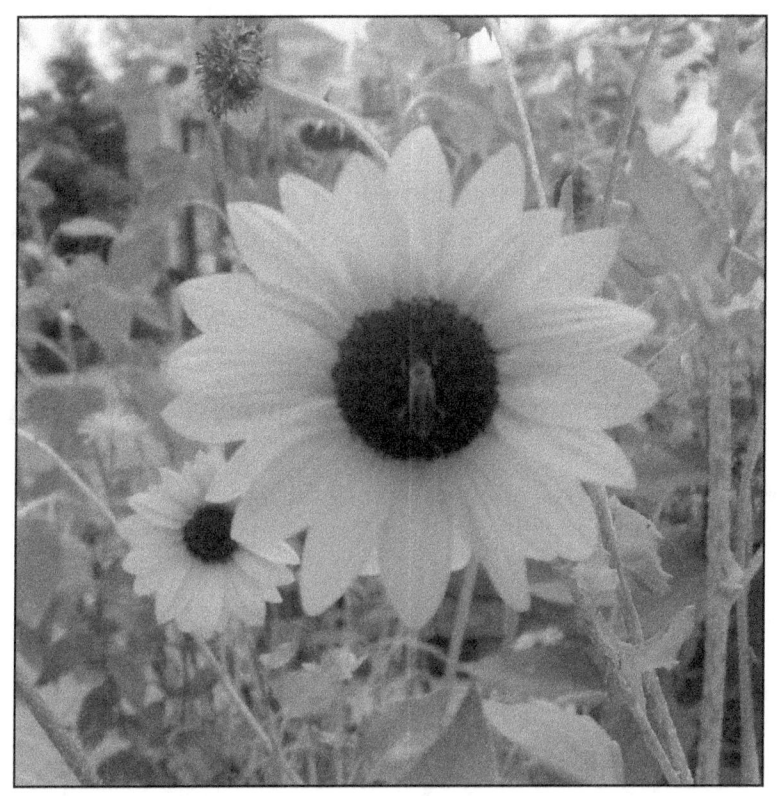

THE END
Our World Goes Round and Round
And in The End
We're in The Ground

•

THE END

Our world goes round and round and in the end, we're unground. In life, we're so busy running around with and maybe attached to sports, shopping, smartphone activities, video games, and work that we forget that we have a limited amount of time left in this world. Thereby need to look into the way we are spending our time on the ground, on this earth, this little ball, before we're placed in the ground and covered with dirt.

•

•

•

•

•

•

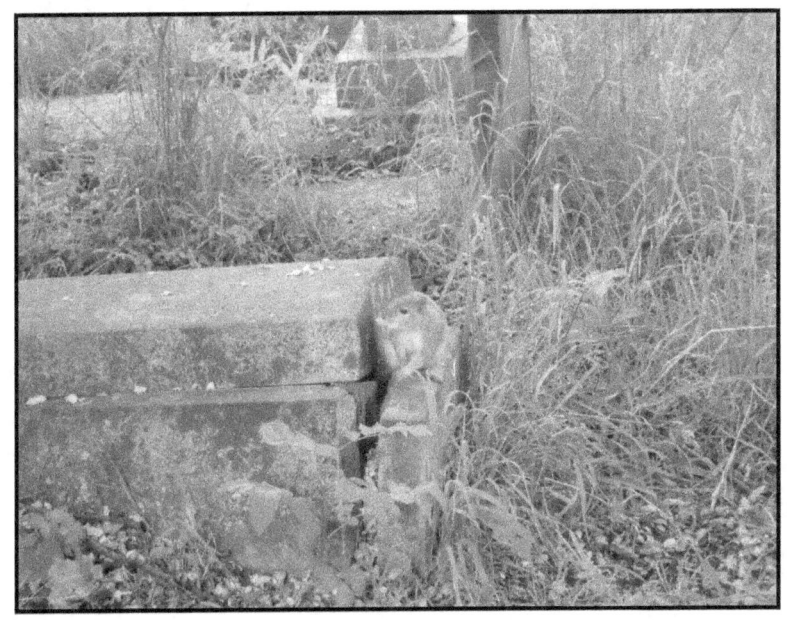

A HOLE

No Matter
Who We Are
or
What We Do
or
Where We Go
We're All Going to
End Up in a Hole

A HOLE

No matter who we are or what we do or even where we go we're all going to one day end up in a hole; you cannot escape the hole.

If you're a golfer and always wanted a hole-in-one well one-day, you'll end up in a hole for one your personal hole in a shiny new casket.

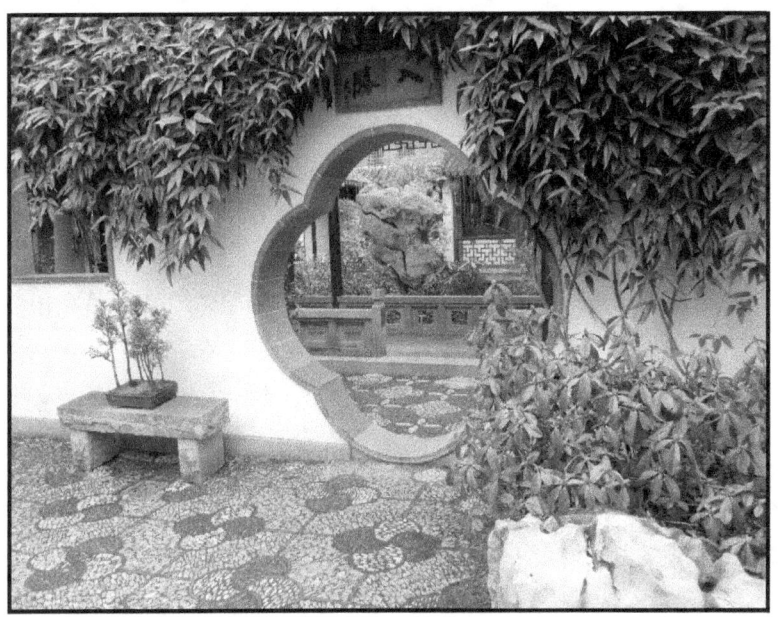

OUR LAST EXPERIENCE

What Will Be Our Last Experience?

Before Death Does Its Clearance

•

OUR LAST EXPERIENCE

What will our last experience be before death does its clearance? Before death clears us out of life, plucks us out of this life. Will we be riding in a car, watching TV, or on vacation when our ultimate experience unfolds? We just don't know if it will be today or tomorrow. So we always need to be ready for our demise and not close our eyes because most of us don't know the place or time it will arise.

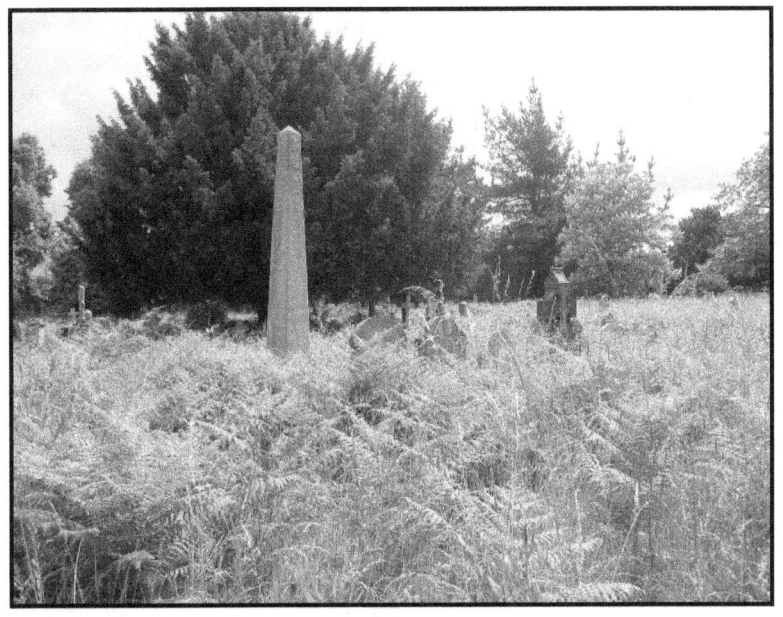

WILL IT MATTER?

All This Fame & Fortune

That We Gathered

At Our End,

Will It Really, Really Matter?

•

WILL IT MATTER?

All this fame and fortune that we gathered, at our end, will it matter? Will any of our accolades, our positions, our possessions or any amount money help us when it's time to go? None of it will be coming with us when we pass on. Even the body we related to life and other earthly bodies with will be left behind. We'll be naked again stripped of all and everything we loved, cherished and clung on to in this world. It's not needed in the next!

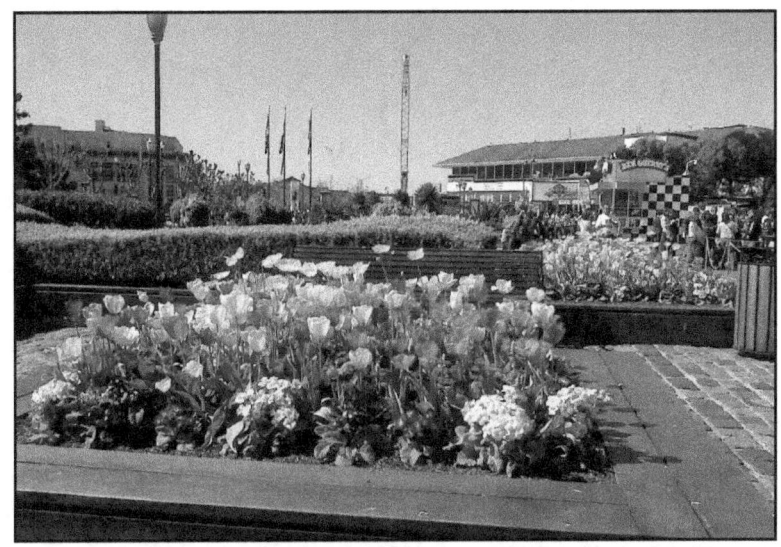

GOT & NOT

We're Never Happy

With What We've Got

We're Always Looking

For What We have Not

●

GOT & NOT

We're never happy with what we've got; we're always looking for what we have not. If we have a dollar, we're looking for two dollars. If we have last year's model car, we want this year's model car. It can be a never-ending cycle of clinging, attachment and accumulation. The relentless quest for more and more, and still more.

Let's open our eyes and not forget, that all this collecting all this more and more will end up with us having no more, when our demise arises.

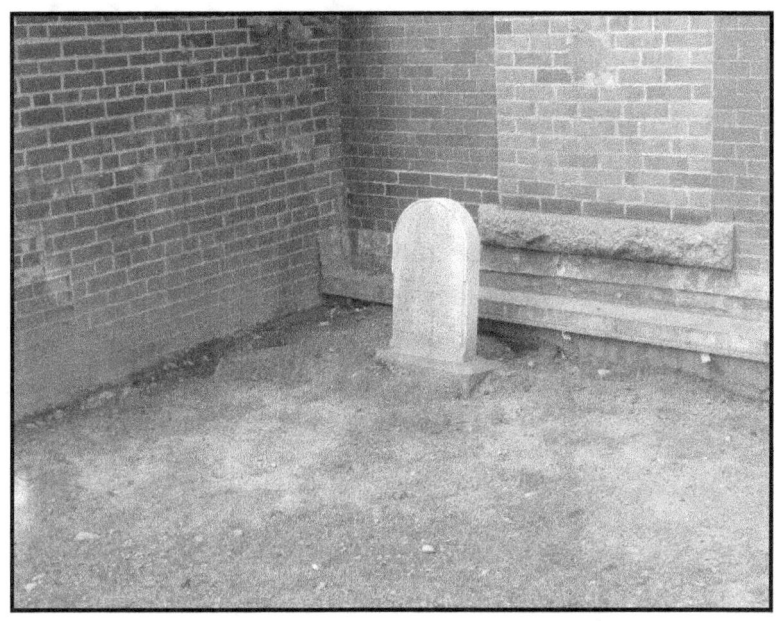

IT IS AMAZING

It's Amazing!

How Permanent

Impermanence Is

•

IT'S AMAZING

It's amazing! How permanent, impermanence is. When we look around we see impermanence in everything, it's all in flux, always changing. Is nothing permanent? The only thing that seems to be permanent in our life is death. One you're dead, you're permanently dead.

•

•

•

•

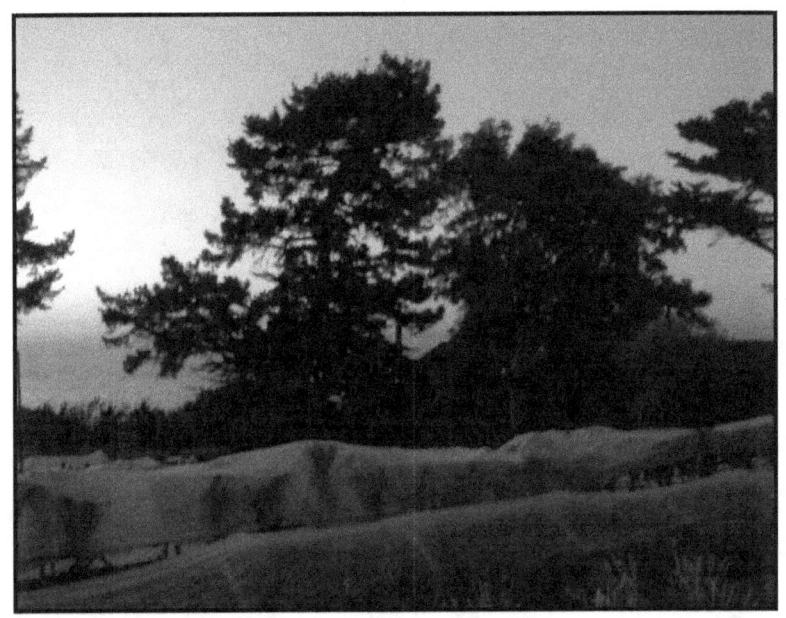

NO SURVIVORS
There Are No
Survivors in Life.

•

NO SURVIVORS

There Are No Survivors in Life. Look around watch the news and you'll see numerous people disappearing, famous and infamous, in-laws and outlaws, friends, foes and family all vanishing before your eyes becoming inanimate forms, corpses to be swept away and buried or burned.

Always remembering that one day someone will be collecting you when your shell empties when your demise arises.

• • •

• • •

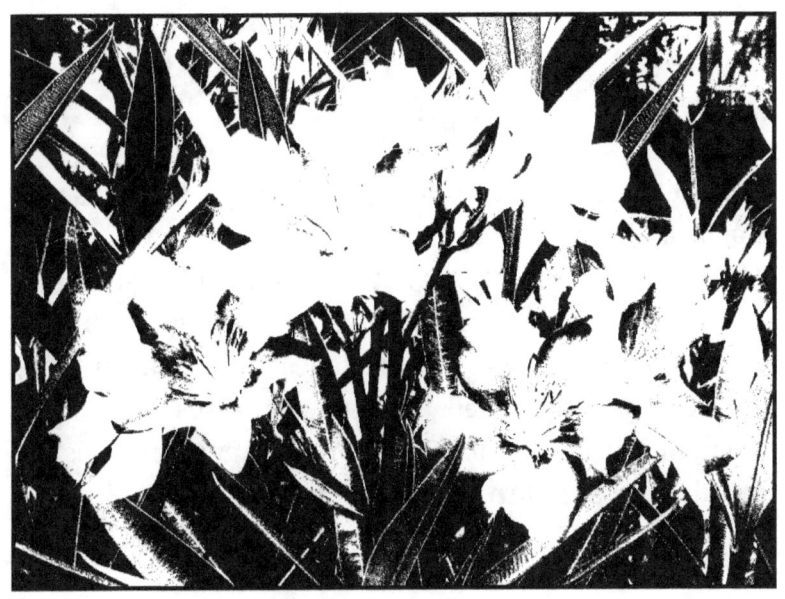

VERY FRAGILE

Life Is Like a Light Bulb

It Has So Many Hours

It's Very Fragile

It Can Break at Any Hour

•

VERY FRAGILE

Life is like a light bulb. It only has so many hours; it's very fragile and can break at any time.

The glass shell is like our outer body the filament is like our inner body. When the light is lite -given life-, it emanating the glow of our existence and has a very long lifespan but the shell that encompasses the light's filament is very fragile and can break at any hour, destroy the filament and turn off the light forever.

•

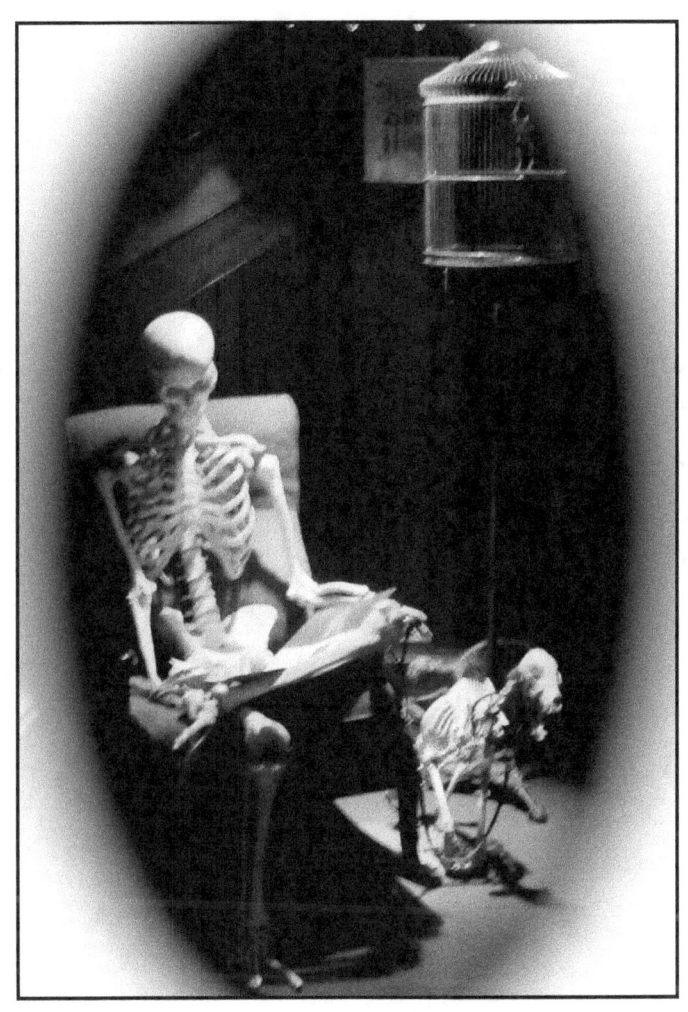

ONE DAY

One Day We'll Retire

One Day We'll Expire

·

ONE DAY

One day we'll retire; one day we'll expire if not expired before we retire. One day we'll go from skin and bones to just bones and from a bag bones to just dust in the wind. When we do expire all that we acquired will no longer be desired or required. Your purse in not required in your hearse.

·

·

·

·

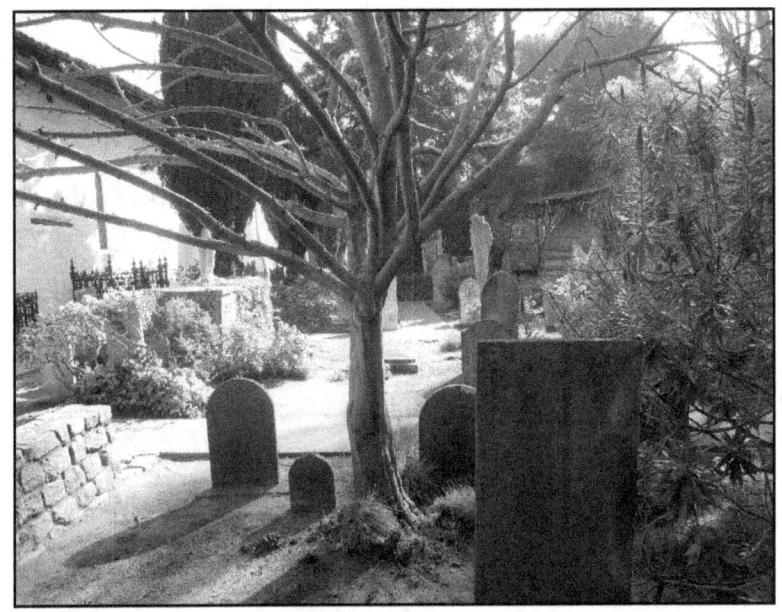

OFF LINE

One Day You're Going Off Line

Your Connection Will Be Severed

You will Be Out of This Life Forever

.

.

•

OFF LINE

One day we will be going along and unexpectedly go offline; our connection severed placing us out of this life forever. One day our connection with this world will be cut, and all our accumulations, all our stuff will be left behind for others to mull over, enjoy, and attach themselves to, then eventually one at a time they too will go offline. They too will be disconnected from their life like all the others who have gone offline before them.

•

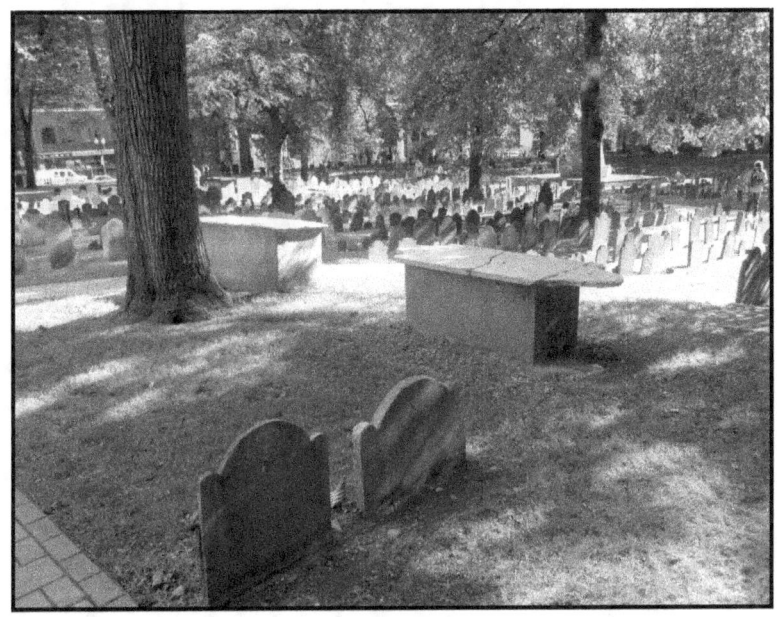

MY COFFIN

My Coffin and Me

When Will We Meet?

Is It Still in The Forest?

Or Displayed

On The Next Street?

•

MY COFFIN

My coffin and me when will we meet? Is it still in the forest or displayed on the next street?

Have you ever wonder if the tree that produces the lumber for your coffin, been cut down yet?

Maybe the box as already been constructed and is on the next street waiting to be filled.

•

•

•

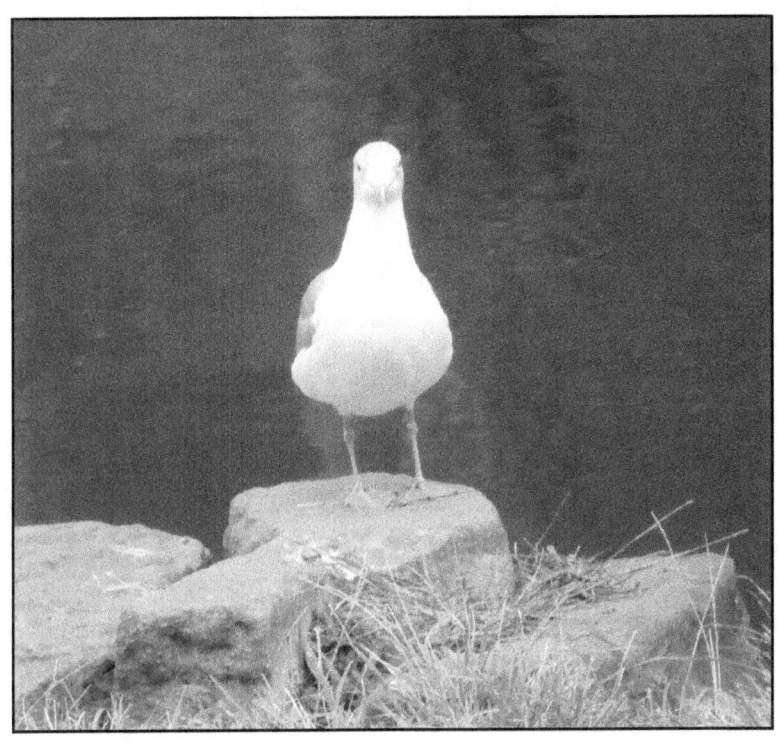

THE GAP

Mind The Gap

Between

Life & Death

•

MIND THE GAP

Mind the gap between life and death. That is the space we are given to live, love and be happy in life. Is the gap being monitored daily? Are you getting as much out of life as you would like or are you just letting time idly pass you by, from day to day as the gap closes and life and death eventually becomes just death and with your demise made ready for the 3Bs? The first B, a black bag to transport you from your last animation point to the second B, the boxing center aka mortuary and finally transferred to your last B, your burial place. A place to rest with all the rest.

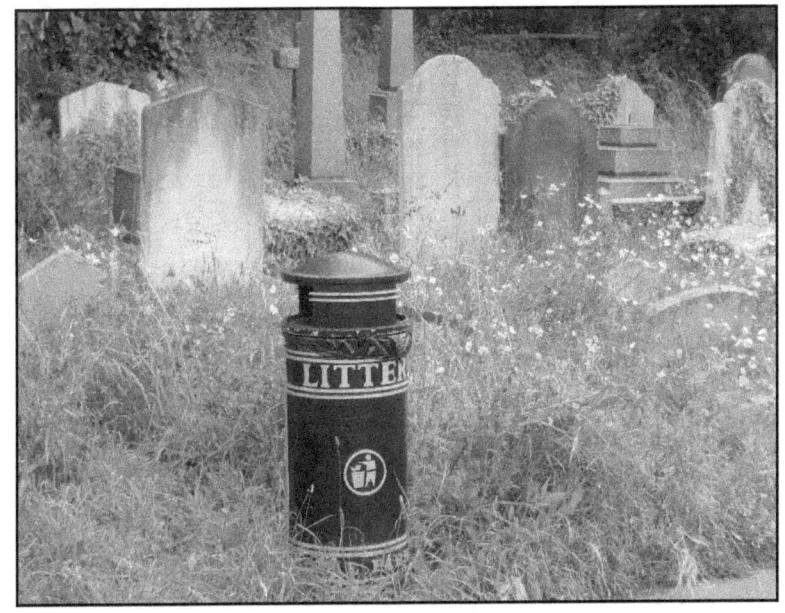

WORRIED

Worried About Losing Everything?

DON'T!

One Day Everything Will Lose You.

•

WORRIED

Worried about losing everything? Don't! One day everything will lose you. Are you concerned about losing any of your accumulations, your so called valuable stuff; all that stuff you gathered and collected over the years? Well, one day all of that will lose you, and everything you hunted and gathered over the years and so worried about will all be distributed. Everything will be sold or given away to others with some of it ending up in the trash, and all of it wiped clean of your worries.

•

•

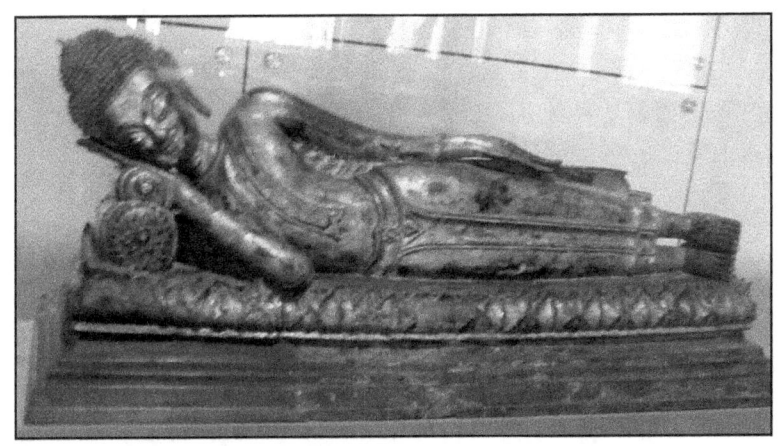

EVERYONE

In The End

Death

Wins Over Everyone

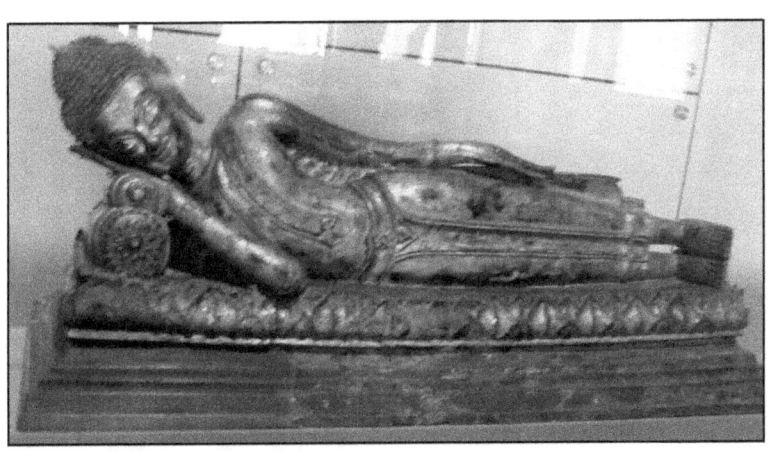

●

EVERYONE

In the end, death will win over everyone. You will not miss out on the death experience. Don't worry one day death will find you wherever you are, then knock on your door, to welcome you aboard.

Will you be ready, prepared or surprise when death arrives?

Your demise could come as a surprise and arise soon after the next sunrise, or it could set in after the next sunset.

●

●

●

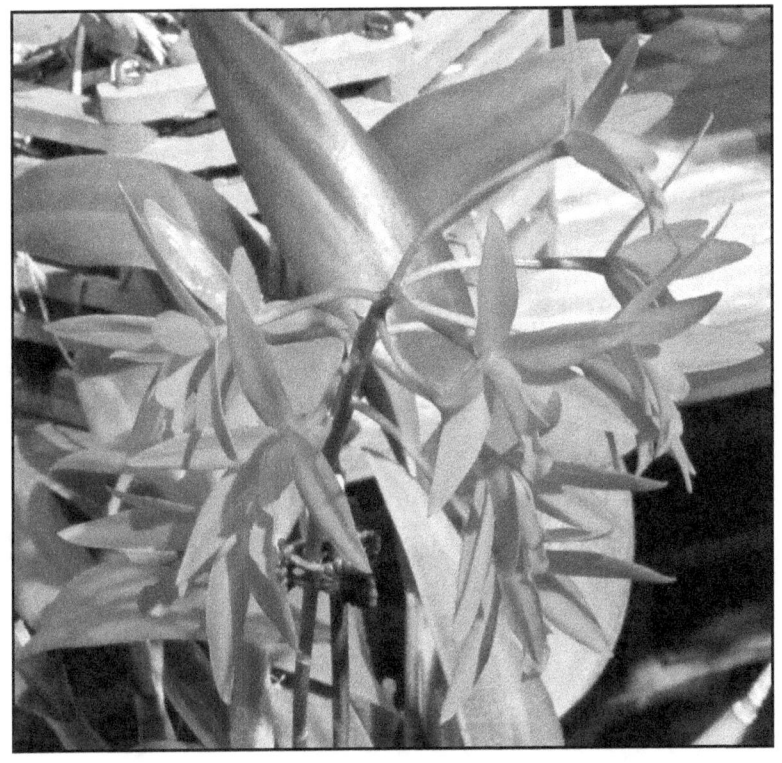

THE TRAVELER

When We Came Out

Of The Womb,

Our Life Was Doomed

And We Started Heading

Toward Our Tomb

•

THE TRAVELER

When we came out of the womb, our life was doomed; a life that came with its twin death. With the conjoined twins life and death in hand, we started heading toward our tomb. And when we arrive at our final destination, when our life gives way to death, will we say what a ride or will we be disappointed and cry?

The Choice is Yours!
You can Make that Decision Right Now!

•   •   •.

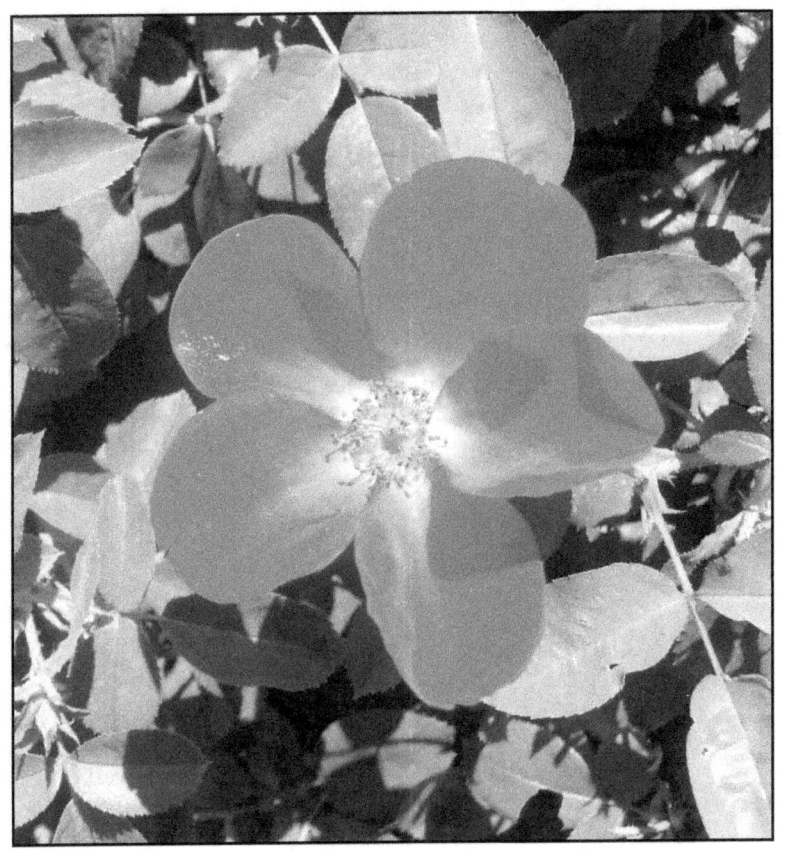

UNDERGROUND

After All of Life's

Ups & Downs,

We'll All End Up

Underground

●

UNDERGROUND

After all of our life's ups and downs, we'll all end up underground. We start on the surface hunting and collecting impermanent worldly things and end up letting them all go when it's time to go down below as a happy or a sad soul with our coffin in tow to be buried in coffin's row.

●

●

●

●

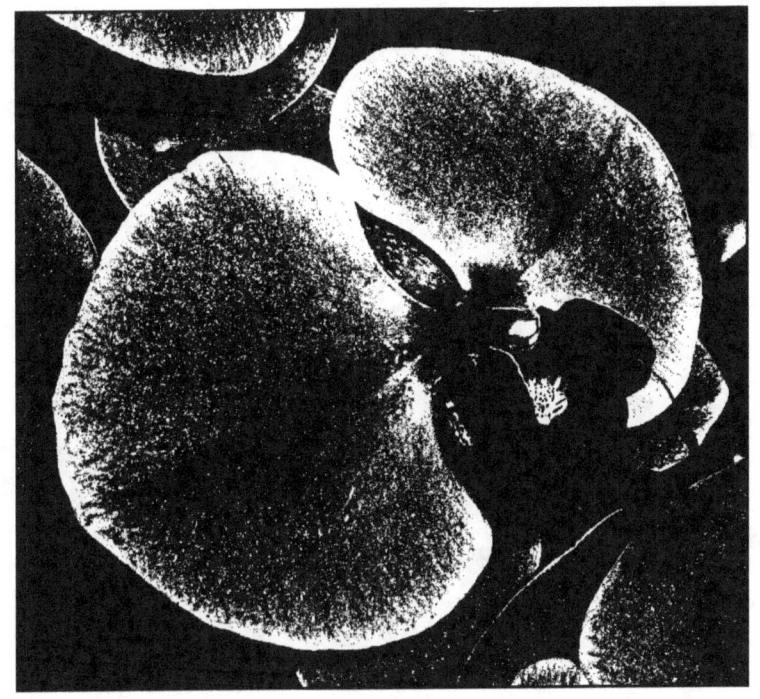

LIFE

LIFE IS LIKE PLAYING

RUSSIAN ROULETTE

THE BULLET IS DEATH

WE SPIN THE CHAMBER

EACH DAY

HOPING THE BULLET

DOESN'T COME UP TODAY

•

•

•

•

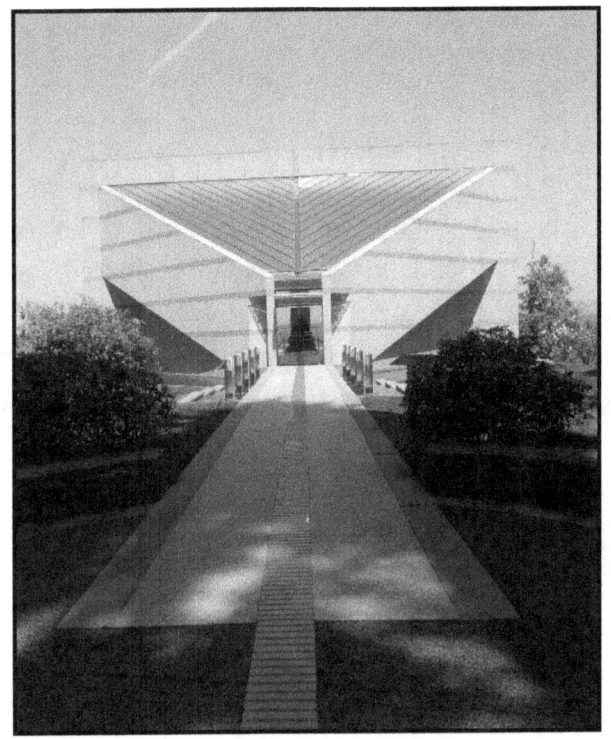

ONE DAY

All Our Accolades

All Our Cash

Everything

We Know & Love

Will One Day Crash

•

ONE DAY

All our accolades, all our cash, everything we know & love will one day crash. Everything we've collected, gathered, worked so hard to obtain, everything we call our own and clung to, care for over our lifetime including our body will all become valueless to us as it is all left behind when our demise arises.

•

•

•

•

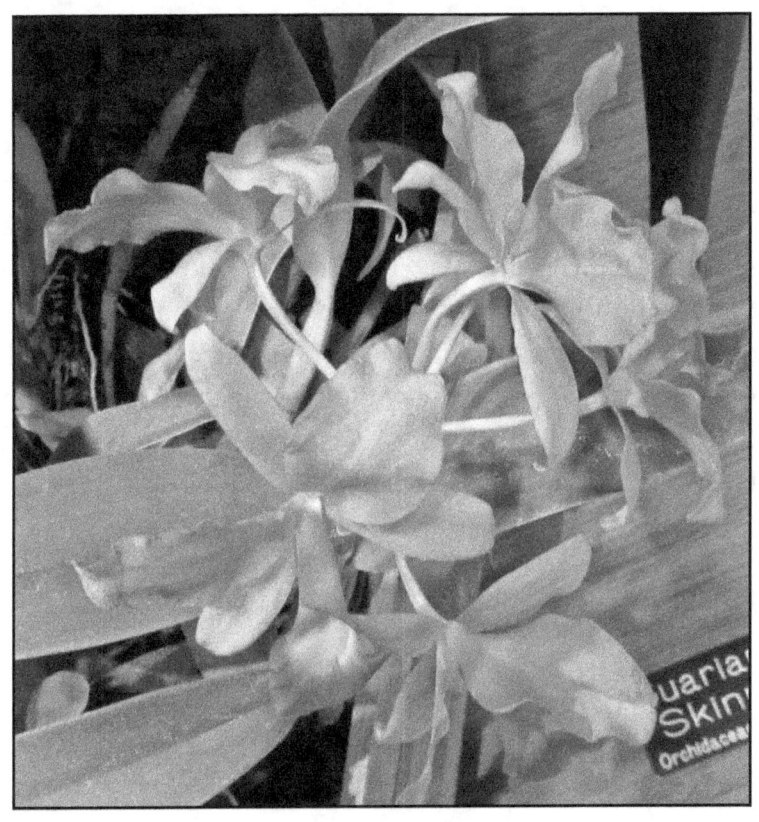

TODAY

Let's Eat, Drink & Be Merry

TOMORROW

We May Be Buried

•   •   •

•

TODAY

Today let's eat, drink and be merry; tomorrow we may be buried. Today is the day to smell the flowers because tomorrow the flowers will be dead. Tomorrow our demise may arise, and we'll be ready to be sized, measured for the box, the coffin for our last presentation that will cause a sensation. A sensation of grief, tears, farewells and some anxiety about the bounty.

•

•

•

•

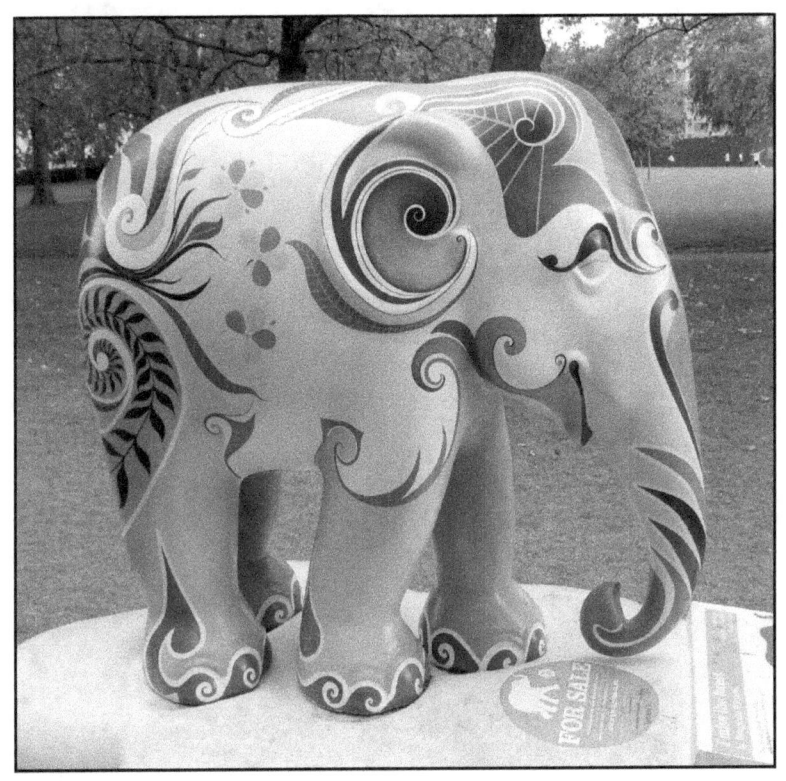

TIME

Not Enough Time for Everything?

Don't Worry!

We'll Always Have Time to Die

•

TIME

Not Enough Time for Everything? Don't Worry! You will Always Have Time to Die. No matter what's going on in your life, putting together a rush project, late for a date, for work, planning a vacation? We must always remember that our demise will override all of it. Our earthly schedules will all vanish, like puffs of smoke on a windy day when death sings its song:
It's time to come along.
This place is where you
no longer belong

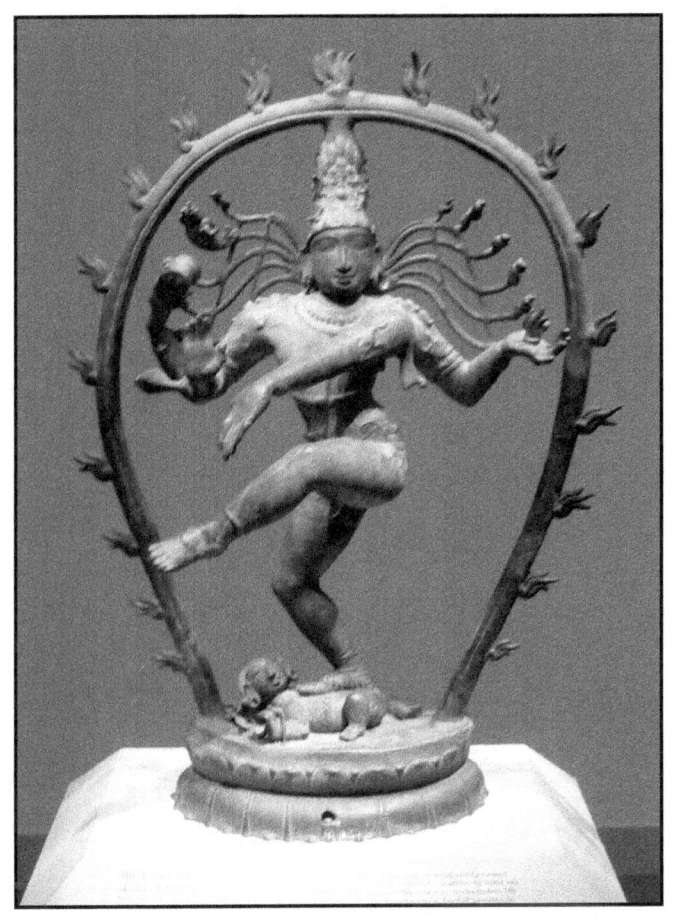

THE CERTIFICATE

Our Birth Certificate

Is Also

Our "Guarantee to Die Certificate"

•

THE CERTIFICATE

Our "Birth Certificate" is also our "Guarantee to Die Certificate," No one will miss out on their last experience in life. No one tells us our Birth Certificate is our Guarantee to Die Certificate when we're young. It's another Fact of Life our parents and educators fail to pass on, probably because their parents and teachers never told them about this most important Fact of Life, the fact that we and everything that surrounds us is impermanent, and we are mortal and will die one day. Our demise time can pop up anywhere, at home, in school, at work, it can arrive at any time and sweep us out of this life.

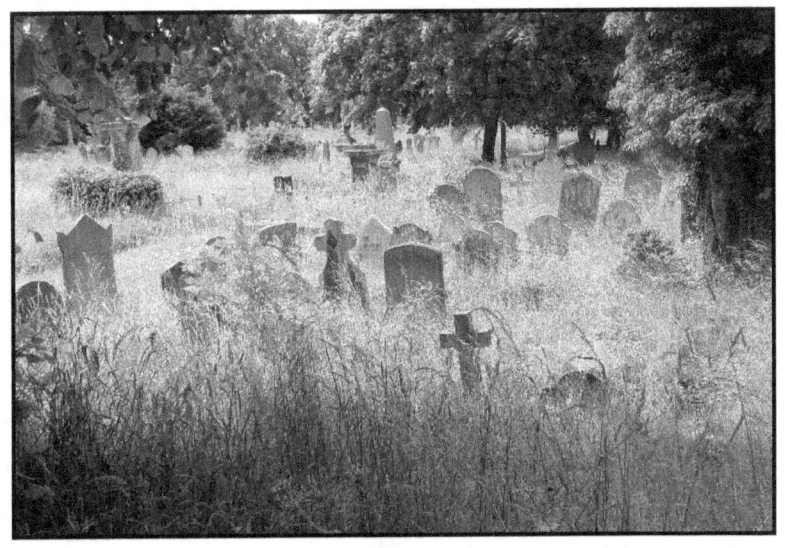

NO ONE

After All Is Said & Done

We'll End Up Being No One

.

.

●

NO ONE

After all is said and done, we will all end up being no one. Look around, read the newspaper, watch TV, go on the internet, or go to a cemetery and see all the graves of people who believed they belonged but now are gone and forgotten. Hopefully, come away with the realization that one day you too will be gone and forgotten. One day you will be just dust in the wind. So seize the day, seize the moment.

Enjoy the day
While it last
Before it turns into your past
or becomes your very last

●

●

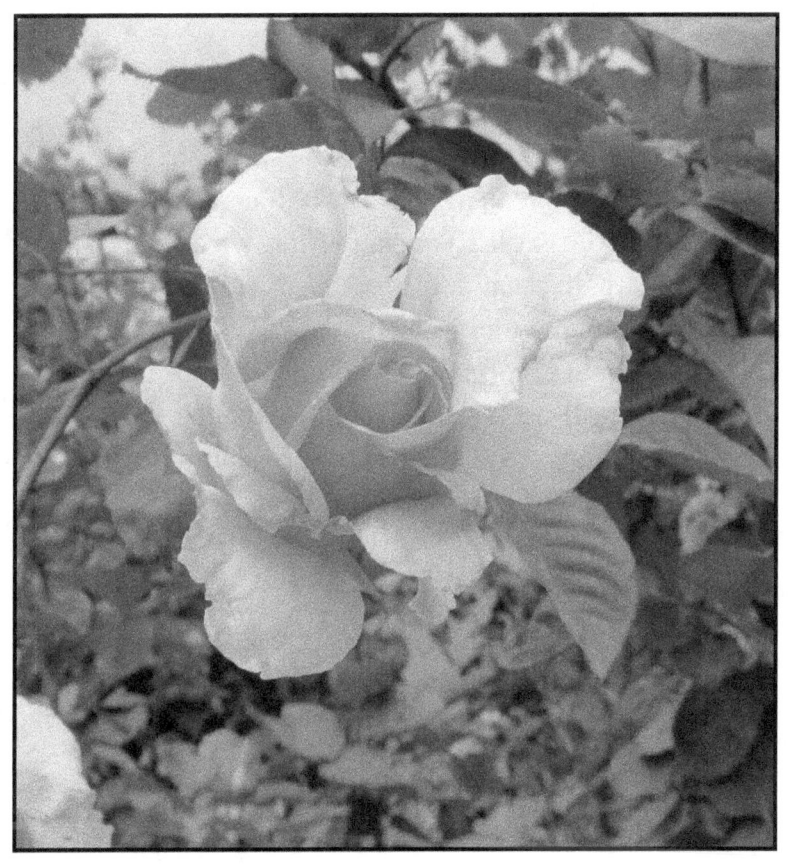

THE GAME OF LIFE
In The Game of Life
Death Is the Final Answer

•

THE GAME OF LIFE

In the game of life, death is the final answer. They don't tell us at birth that life is a game, and we are all players, players with likes and dislikes, with our ups and our downs, with needs and wants.

We are all game pieces that will one day not be needed, pieces that will be removed from the game of life when the piece is, worn out or broken and declared dead.

•

•

•

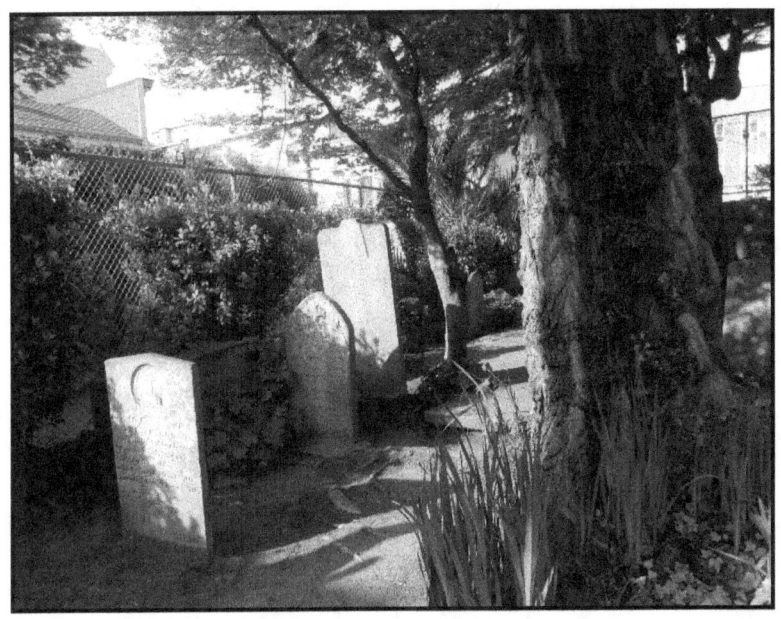

AFTER WE'RE GONE

The World Got Along

Before We Were Born

And It'll Get Along

After We're Gone

•

AFTER WE ARE GONE

The world got along before we were born and it will get along long after we're gone. Look at history and see how many others there were who believed they were so strong, and belonged, or others who have thought themselves indispensable, but after they passed on the world got along and moved on without them.

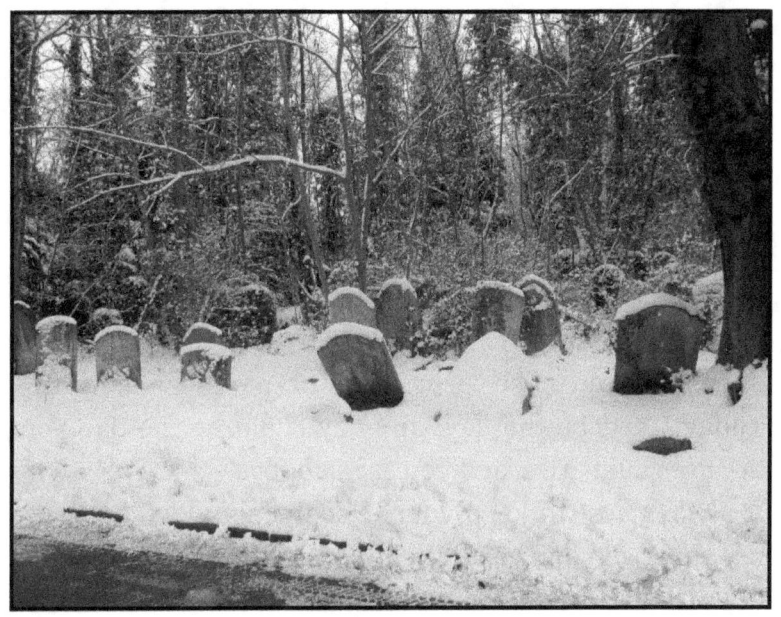

TODAY

It Could Be Over

By The End of The Day

Oh Me, Oh My!

I Just Might Die Today

•

•

TODAY

It could be over by the end of the day. Oh me, oh my! I just might die today. Today could be the day your demise arises. Would you be surprised or prepared if it arrived?
Today could be the day; any day could be the day your demise could arise, and you say goodbye.
It always best to keep your eyes open, be prepared and not surprised for the day death comes by and says: Hi.

•

•

•

•

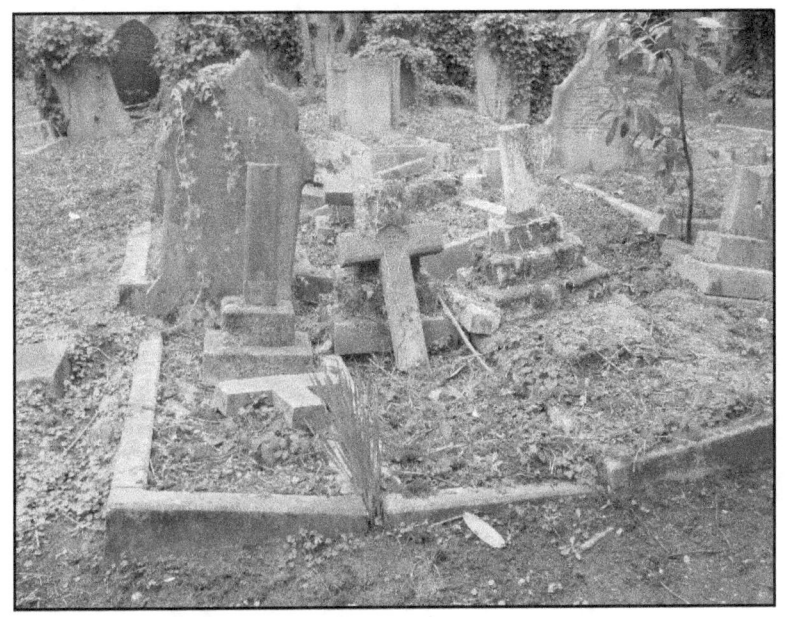

DEATH

No Matter What Kind of Life

We Lead, Or Not Lead

One Day, Death

Will Bring Us

To Our Knees

•

Will Our Life End Today?
Or!
Will We Be Given Another Day?

•

•

•

•

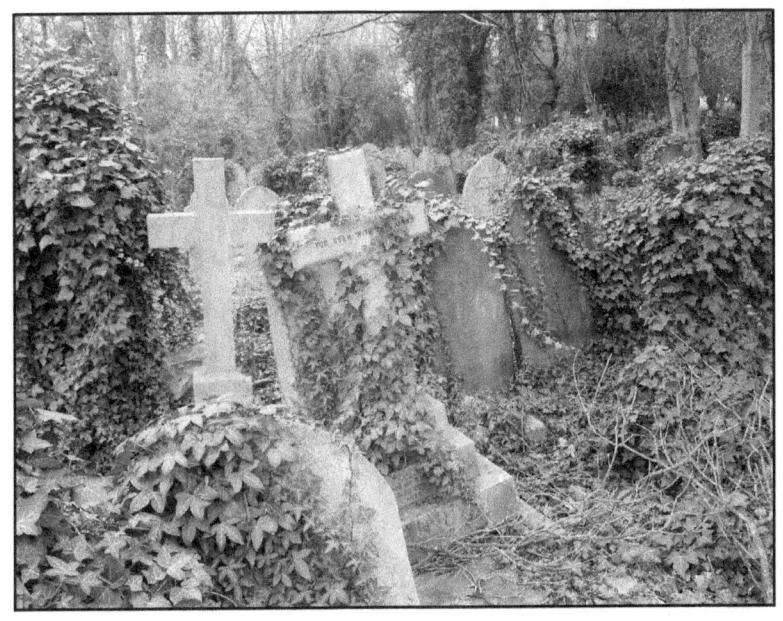

MY LIFE, YOUR LIFE
I Have My Life,
You Have Yours
We're Both Going to Die
That's for Sure

•

•

MY LIFE, YOUR LIFE

I have my life; you have yours. What we all have in common is we were both born and one day we are going to die; that's for sure. When will it happen? Most of us do not know. It could be Later Today, Tomorrow, next week or next year. Will we be ready or surprised when our demise arises? It's up to you, and me, to prepared ourselves for the occasion, the time death comes by and says: Hi!

•

•

•

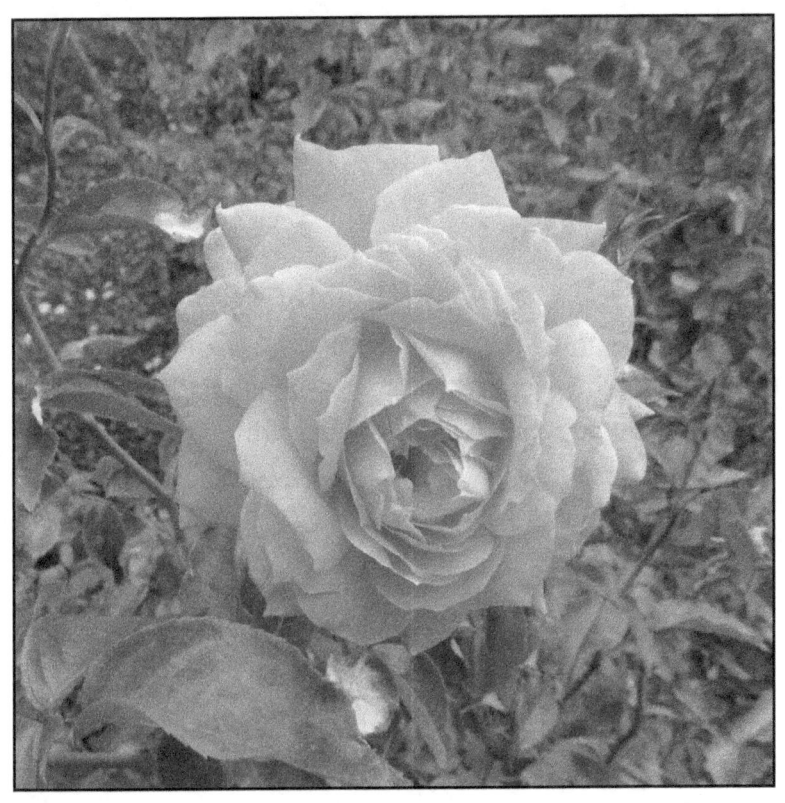

AT ANYTIME

Death May Show Up

When We Least Expect It.

•

•

AT ANYTIME

Death is going to show up when we least expect it.
Will you be prepared or surprised when it arrives?
Will you be ready or will you ask why? Why? Why?

•   •   •

•

•

•

•

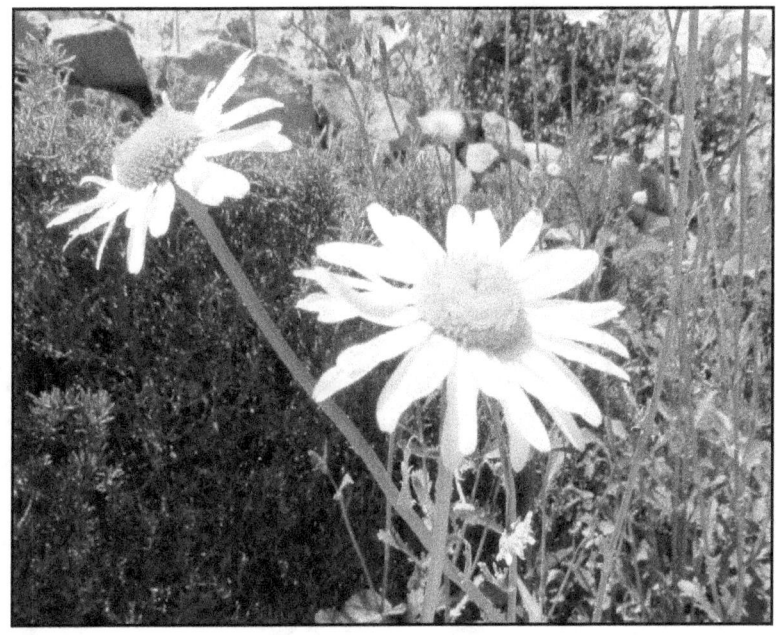

ONE DAY

We Work So Hard

We Gain So Much

Then One Day

Death Clears It All Away

•

•

ONE DAY

We work so hard we gain so much then one-day death sweeps it all away. All of our family, our friends, our accolades and all our money will be left behind when our demise arises and looks us in the eye and says: Hi!

•

•

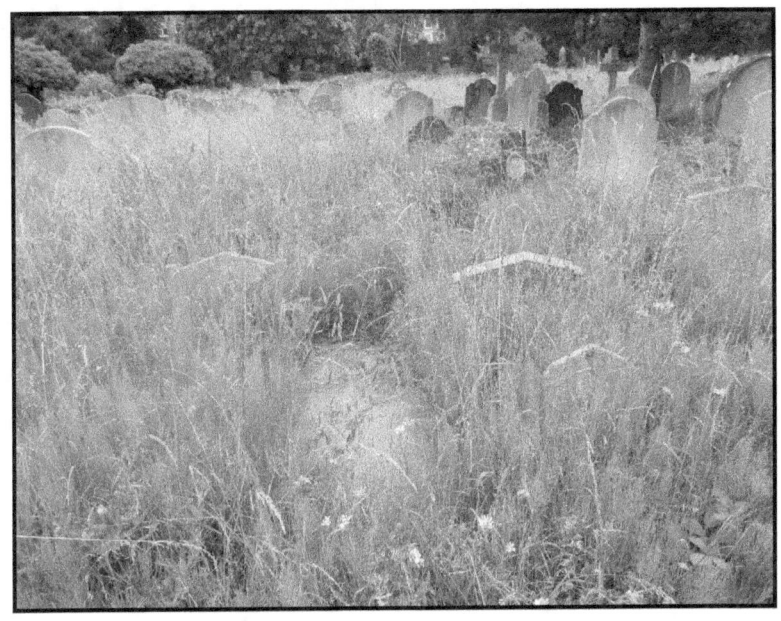

TIME

- Weeks Go By
- Months Go By
- Years Go By
- And Every Day
- We Get Closer
- And Closer, And Closer
- To The Day We Die

•

•

TIME

Days, weeks, months, and years go by and every day we get closer, and closer, and closer, to the day we die. The day our demise arrives and look us in the eye, and says Hi, you're my guy.

Time is just slipping by so fast and turning into our past. How long will it last? We don't know.

Now's the time to tune-in to what time we may have left, and take the time we have now, to live, love, and be happy.

•   •   •

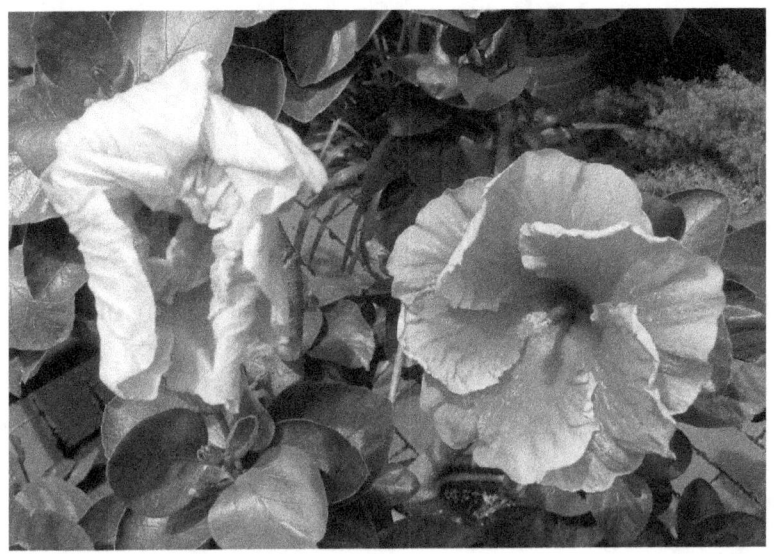

PERFORMANCE

One Day Our Form

Will Cease to Perform

•

•

•

THE PERFORMANCE

One day our form will cease to perform. One day our form will break down and die, and the curtain will come down on our performance, our last act. Our time on life's stage will be over. All the costumes and props we used in life will be given away to others, to use in their performances. After we leave, the curtain will rise again, and the show will go on, without us, like it went on before us, before being cast, in our performance on life's stage.

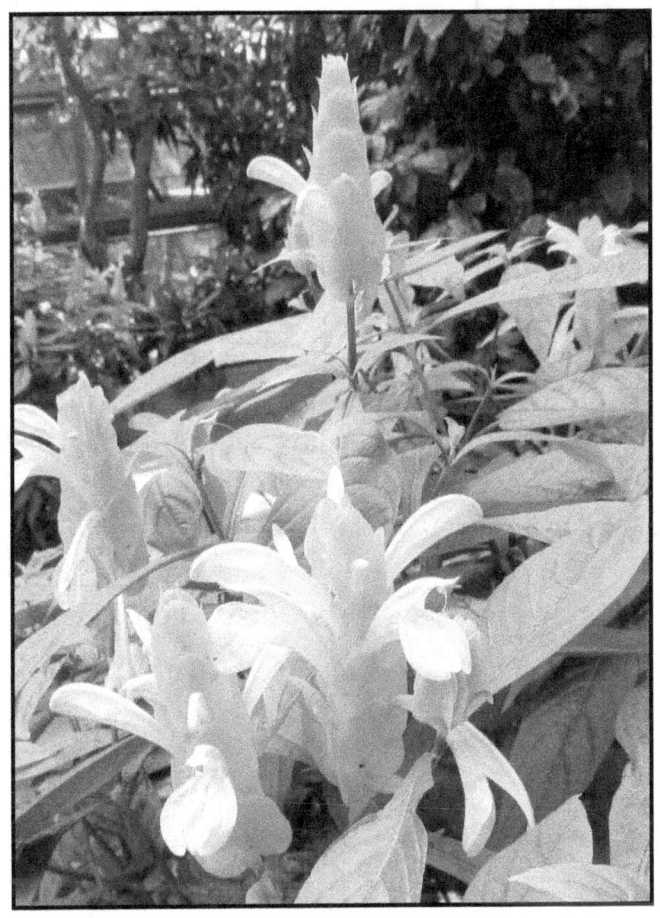

INTERESTED

If We're Interested in Living

We Have to Be Interested in Dying

•

•

INTERESTED

If we're interested in living, we have to be interested in dying. Our impending death can be a catalyst for living a fuller life. Knowing that our time here is limited, and our departure date is unknown can help elucidate how little time we may have left on this speck of dust, we call earth. Death can show us how to live and wake us up to our limited time, the time we need to cherish before we perish.

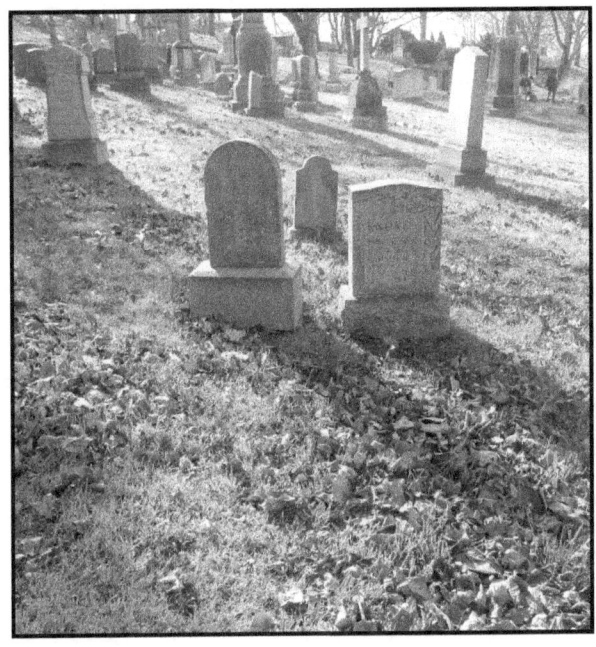

CHOICE

No Matter What Kind of Life
We Choose, Or Not Choose,
Or Can't Choose
We'll All End Up in a Place,
We Don't Choose; **DEAD**

•

•

CHOICE

No matter what kind of life we choose, or not choose, or can't choose we'll all end up in a place, we don't choose: Dead. The endgame in life is death. If we remember that, then we can begin to live a clearer and brighter life, a life free of the fear of our demise.

•

•

•

•

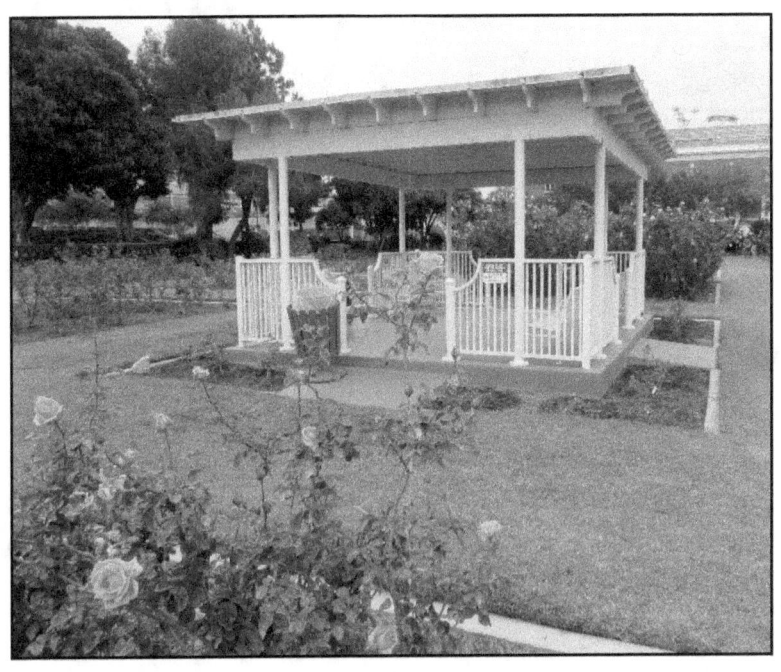

DON'T GET ATTACHED

Don't Get Attached Today,

Cause One Day

You'll Have to Break Away

The Stronger the Glue

The More You'll Feel Blue

•

•

DON'T GET ATTACHED

Don't get attached today, cause one day you'll have to break away. The stronger the glue, the more you'll feel blue. The more attached you are to life and its trappings the more painful it will be for you and everyone close to you when your demise arises.

•

•

•

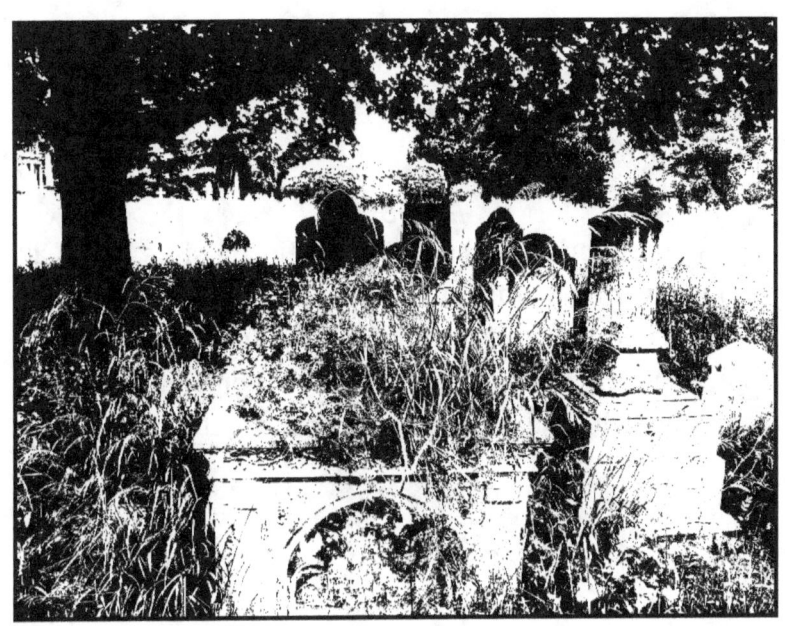

IN ALL SIZES

Big, Small

Short, Tall

They Make

Coffins in Sizes

For Us All

•

•

ALL SIZES

Big, small, short, tall, they make coffins in sizes for us all. You'll never be too big or too small for a coffin. They have all sizes and are ready and waiting for someone's demise to arise and order a casket or an urn. Remember one day someone will order one for your final event.

•

•

•

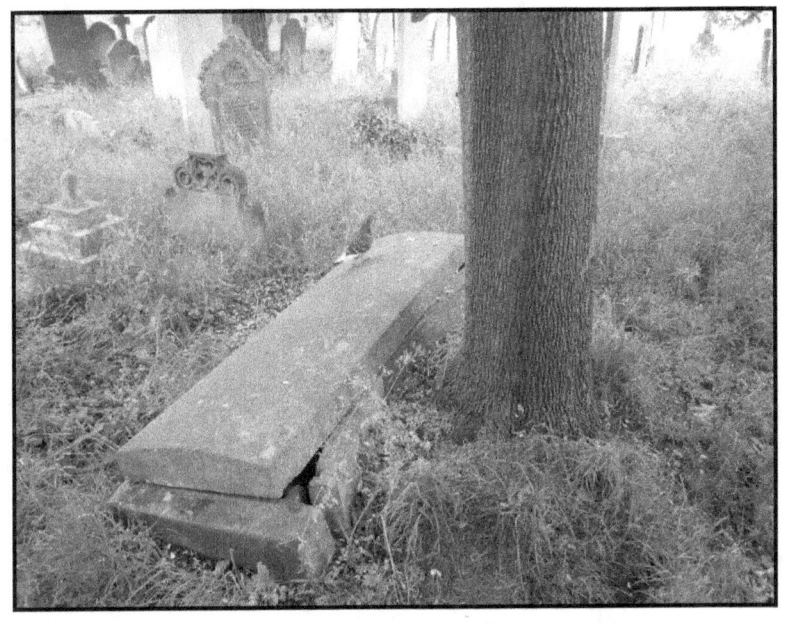

A GRAVE

No Matter Who We Are
Or What We Do
There's a Grave
Waiting for Me & You

• • •

•

•

A GRAVE

No matter who we are, or what we do, there's a grave waiting for you and me. Our form in a box aka coffin, disposed of, under some dirt, in a cemetery with a headstone over our head, or as ashes in an urn on a shelf near someone's bed.

•

•

•

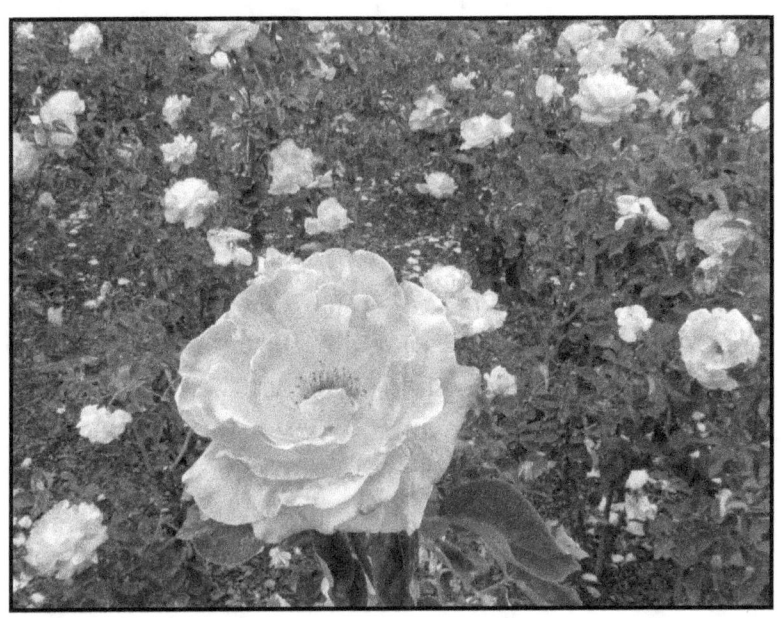

OUR DAY WILL COME
Someone Dies Every Day
One Day It will Be Our Day

•

•

•

OUR DAY WILL COME

Someone dies every day; one day it'll be our day to die. One day it will be our turn to say goodbye, Adios, Hasta la Vista baby, I won't be coming back. Our turn to leave it all behind, everything we clung to over the years: our likes, our dislikes, our ups and downs, our past, our future and all our other worldly trapping.

•

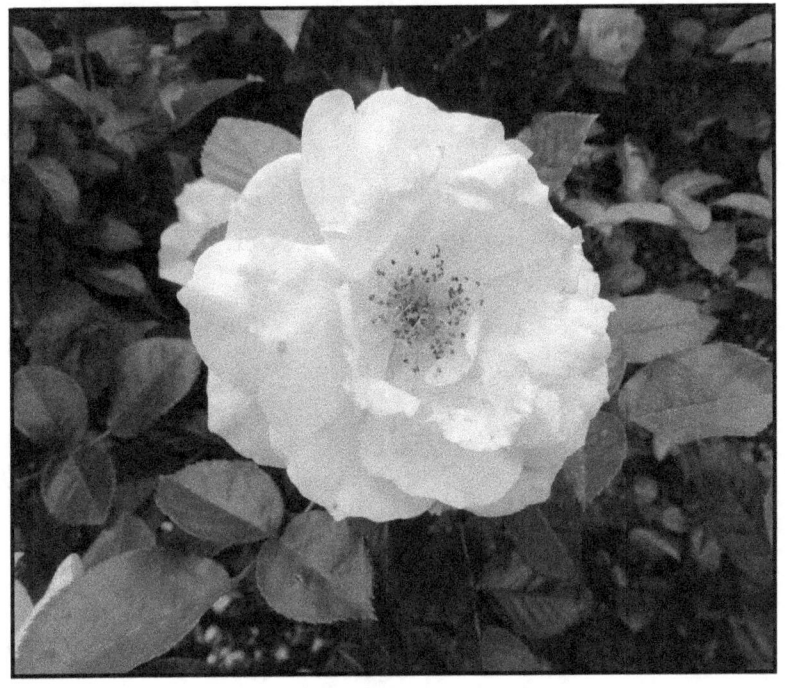

EVERY DAY'S A BIG DAY

Every Day's A Big Day

If We're Alive

And If We're Not

We Won't Sweat It

•

•

EVERY DAY'S A BIG DAY

Every day's a big day if we're alive, and if we're not, we won't sweat it. Corpses don't sweat.

So let's make today a big day, let's make every day a big day while we're alive by remembering: that tomorrow we could be dead.

•

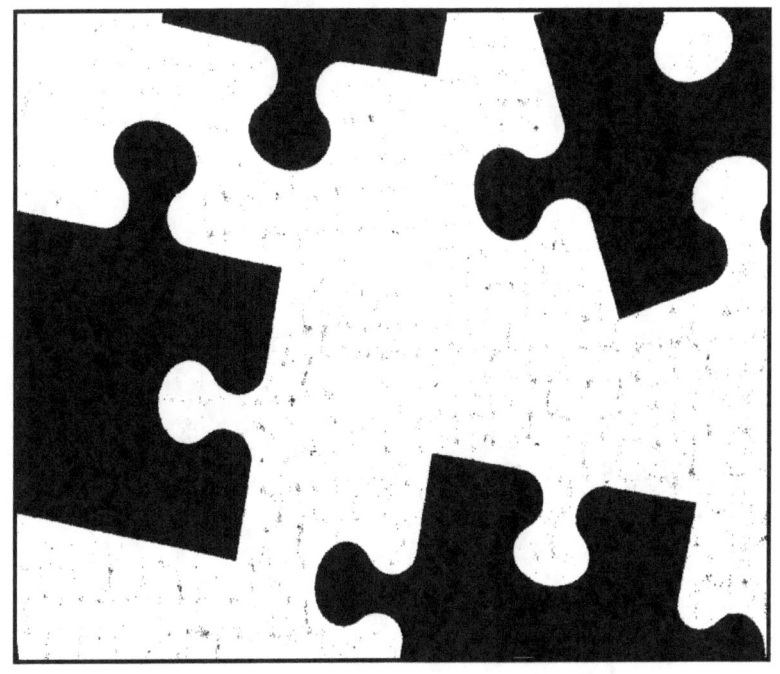

24

In The Next 24

We Could End Up

Being No More.

•

•

24

In the next 24, we could end up being no more! Will we have the next 24 or will we be taken sometime B4? We just can't be sure we will pass thru the next 24 and get any more 24s, or maybe taken sometime B4 our current 24 ends.

•

•

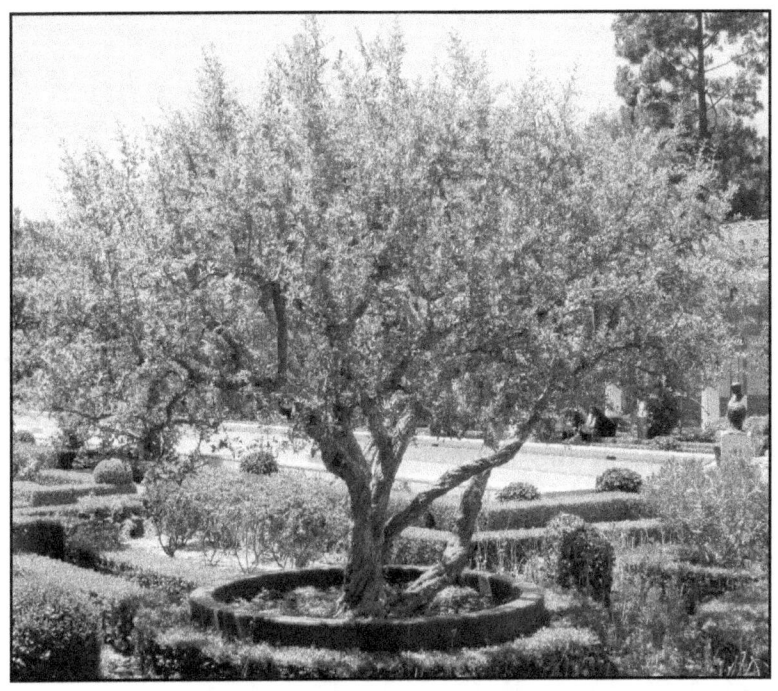

AT ANY TIME

Plan Your Week
But Keep in Mind
That Death Can Happen
At Any Time

•

•

AT ANY TIME

Plan your week but keep in mind that death can happen at any time. It can happen to any of us in any day of the week, at any time of the day or night, at any place we might be, in the morning, afternoon, or evening. At a movie show, or on the road, death will find us if it's our time to go.

•

•

•

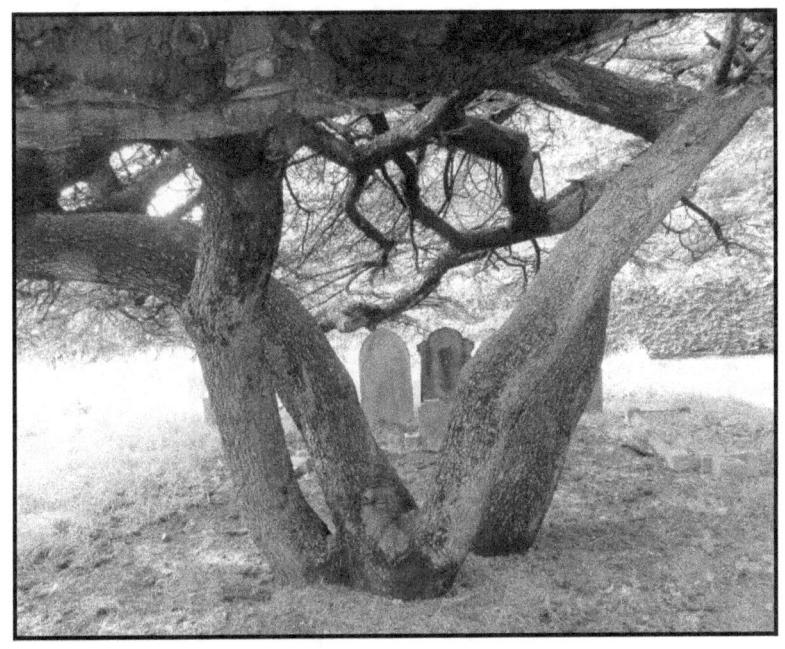

NEVER AGAIN

One Day We Will Be Going Along

And Death Will Ring Its Gong

We'll Sing Our Last Song

And Never Again Belong

.

.

NEVER AGAIN

One day we will be going along, and death will ring its gong, we'll sing our last song, and never again belong. One day our demise will arise, and our belonging days will subside, death will say Hi, and we will say goodbye to the sun and the sky.

.

.

.

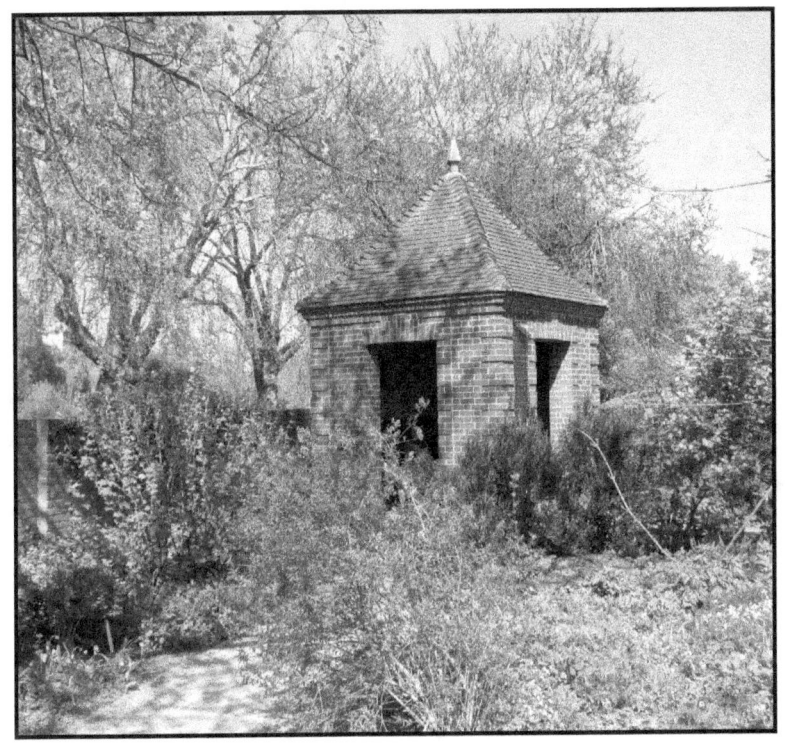

ANYMORE

In A Fancy Coffin

Or On a Slab in The Morgue

We Won't Be Walking

Or Talking Anymore

•

ANYMORE

In a fancy coffin, or on a slab in the morgue, we won't be doing any walking or talking anymore. Our time will be over, our body not alive and everything we had before our demise, nullified.

•

•

•

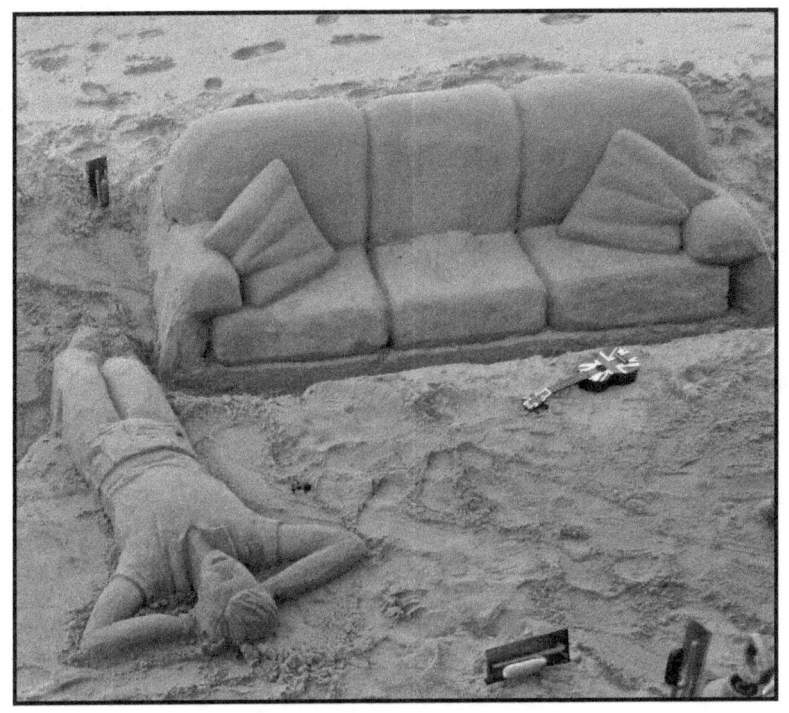

A VANISHING ACT

We're All Magicians And

One-Day We'll Perform

A Vanishing Act

.

.

A VANISHING ACT

We're all magicians, and one-day we'll perform a vanishing act, and disappear from this life with no purse, and no baggage in hand, and return to the land of nonexistence.
You won't Need Your Purse
In Your Hearse

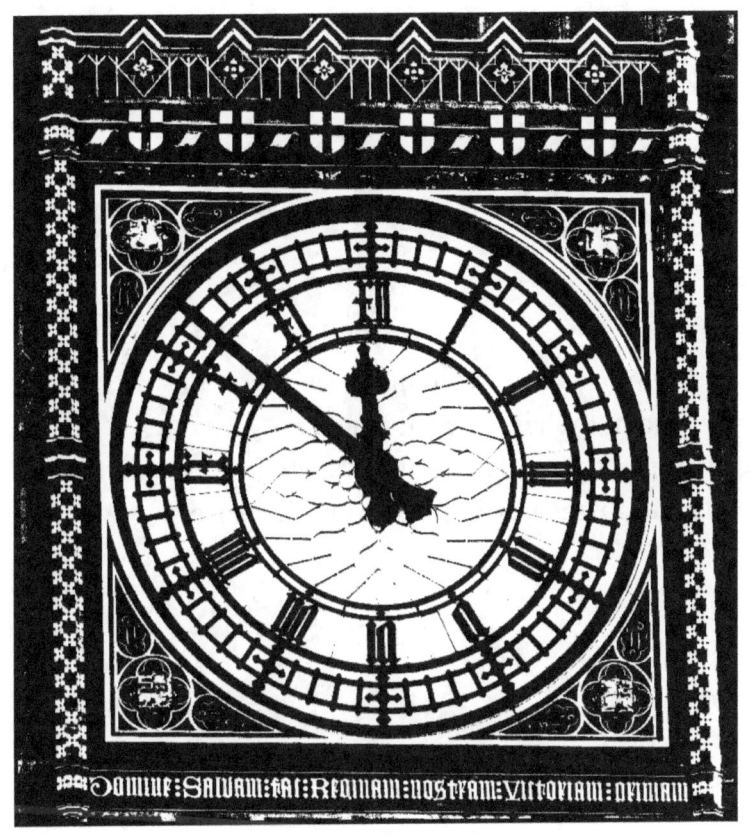

TIME

At The Time of Our Demise

It Won't Be What We've Collected

But What We've Given Up

•

•

TIME

At the time of our demise, it won't be what we've collected but what we've given up.

If we are wise and gave it all up before our demise, we will have a peaceful, happy ending surprise.

•

•

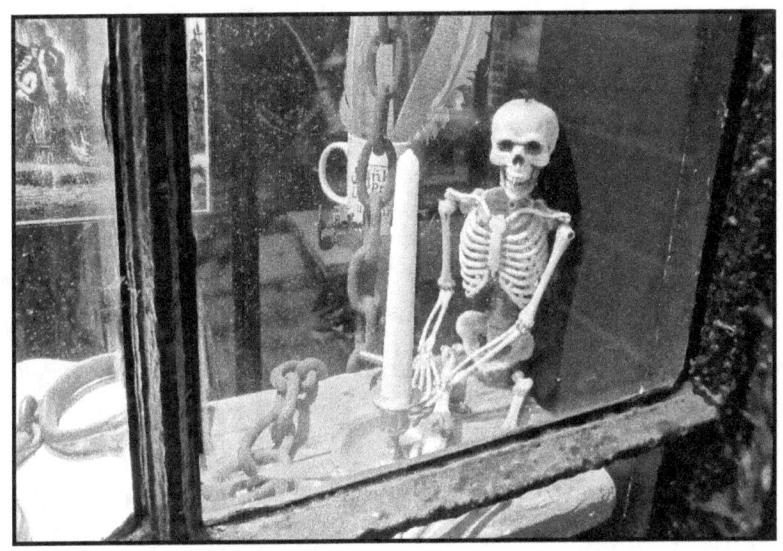

3 B's

One day we'll get the three B's

Bagged, Boxed and Buried

.

.

.

•

•

3 B's

One day it will be time, for the three B's; to be: Bagged, Boxed, and Buried. When our form ceases to perform we will encounter our first "B," when they collect us and put our corpse in a black plastic bag, -first "B"- for transport, to our second "B" the boxing center aka mortuary. At the funeral home, we will be made ready for our last exhibition: where we will be the guest of honor at our last Wake. Then after the Wake ends transported to our last "B" event: our burial.

•

•

•

•

"The End"

The Book Is Over
And We're at The Last Page
One Day Our Life Will Be Over
And We'll Be in Our Last Stage

.

.

.

.

SEIZE THE DAY

Enjoy The Day While It Last
Before It Turns into Your Past
Enjoy The Day; Run and Play
Cuz It Could Be Your Final Day

• ECHOES FROM THE PAST •
Can You Hear Them?

Oh, how small a portion of earth will hold us when we are dead, who ambitiously seek after the whole world while we are living!

Philip II of Macedon, (382–336 B C)

•

"Remembering that you are going to die is the best way I know to avoid the trap of thinking you have something to lose. You are already naked. There is no reason not to follow your heart."

Steve Jobs, (1955 - 2011)

•

"If I had my life to live over again, I would form the habit of nightly composing myself to thoughts of death. I would practice, as it were, the remembrance of death. There is not another practice, which so intensifies life. Death, when it approaches, ought not to take one by surprise. It should be part of the full expectancy of life."

Muriel Spark (1918-2006)

•

•

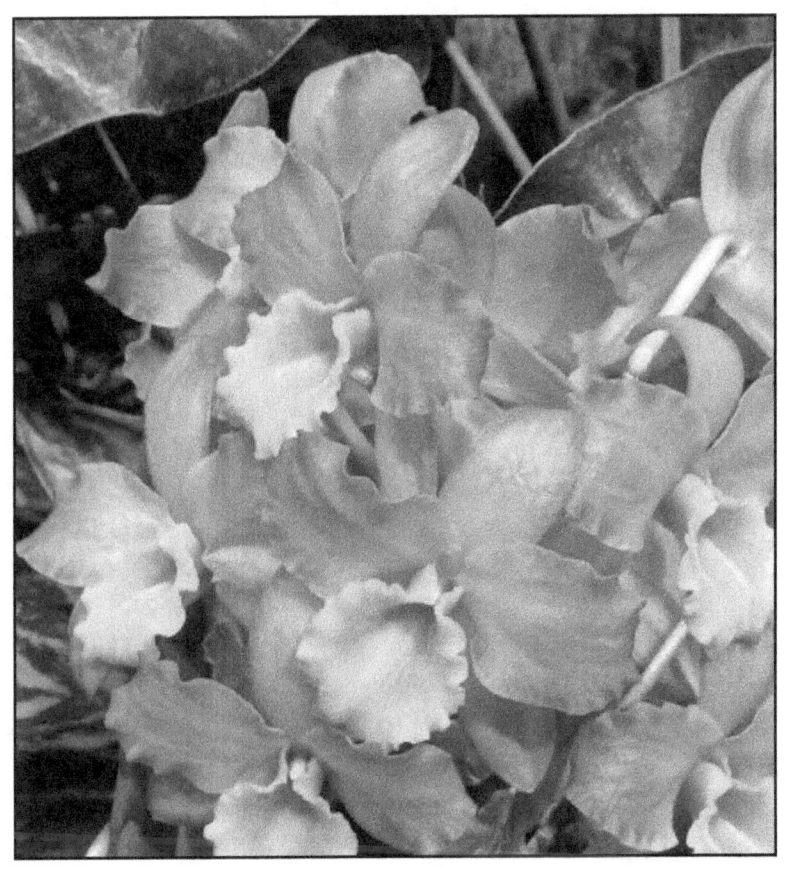

YOUR DEMISE WILL ARISE

YOUR DEMISE WILL ARISE

Our life arose, so our death will arise too. We were born, and we will die. Death is like a huge elephant that sits on us and never gets up. When will our demise arise and will we be ready for it? Who knows? Most of us try not to think about it; some people's attitude is to drink-to-forget because not thinking about it might make it go away. Others try pushing it out of their mind by putting their life in fast-forward and filling their days with time-consuming activities like sports, shopping, parties, eating, going online and numerous other activities. What kind of life are we living: if we exclude the biggest and most important part of our living experience? If we exclude the part that will one-day sweep everything away: all our friends, our family, our money, all our stuff, and all the other experiences we have collected over the years. All that will all be nullified by our demise.

Death will arise and catch up to us one day. It's getting closer and closer with each passing day. It's like a hungry tiger stalking its prey waiting for the right time to strike and consume.

•

•

•

•

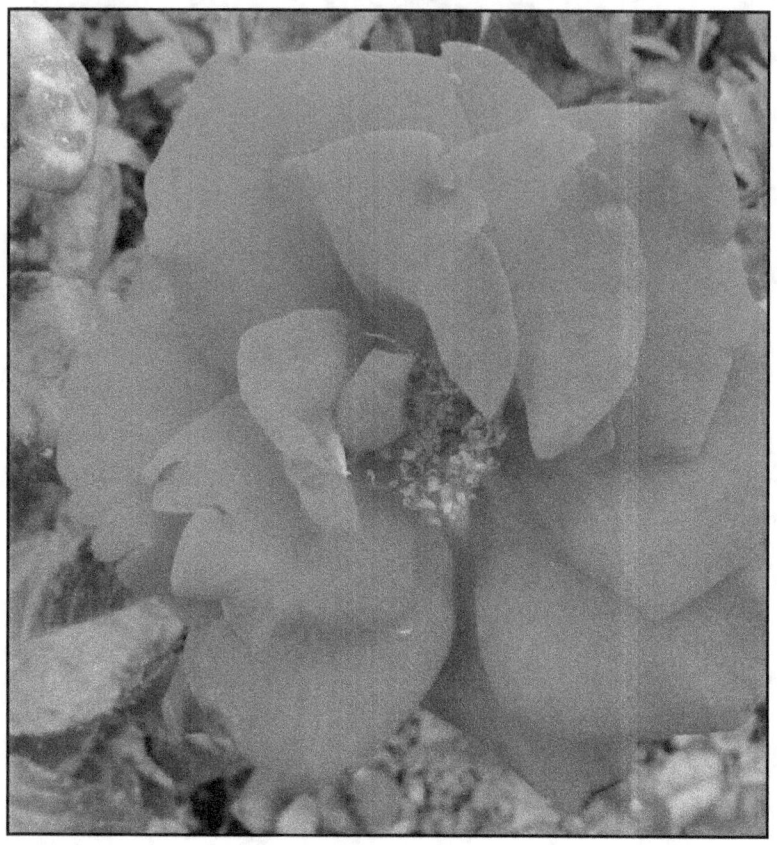

BIRTH AND DEATH

Our birth certificate is also our guarantee to die certificate. There's no getting away from it. Death is a crucial part of our living experience, and its awareness needs to be with us all the time. Death needs to be our common denominator for everything we do in this life, thereby dividing all of our daily experiences by the fact that we'll die one day, and today could be that day. We'll die like all the other people who have died before us.

With the awareness that we could die at any time and everyone we know could die at any time too. It seems prudent to realize that we need not bear any ill feeling toward anyone, especially ourselves since we only have this moment and this moment alone, so why, waste it, being anything else but positive. Our next moment is tentative. Even though death may be just around the corner and we don't know what corner and most of us never will. Our demise could arise in the next 5 minutes, 5 hours, five days, five years, or maybe in 25 years. It's like a time bomb ticking away, and we don't know when it'll explode and discharge us from this life. Are we ready for it, prepared to go at any time, whether we're in rain or snow, or in sun or shade?

We need to remember our demise will arise one day so let's keep our eyes open and prepared for it.

BE PREPARED

NOT SURPRISED

WHEN DEATH ARRIVES

A SIMPLE GAME

Life Is a Simple Game

There Are No Winners

There Are No Losers

Everyone Comes Away from It

Like They Came into It: Naked

LIFE: NAKED IN; NAKED OUT

Music & Movies

- Music you may enjoy:
  "Life is Just a Bowl of Cherries"
  Performed by: Johnny Mathis
  "Dust in the Wind"
  Performed by: Kansas
  "Enjoy Yourself"
  Performed by: Guy Lombardo
- Movies you may enjoy:
  "Harold and Maude"
  "Hereafter"
  "Joe Black"

* * * * * * * * * *

ENJOY LIFE

Enjoy Life

It's later then you think

Enjoy Life

You may be on the brink

Enjoy Life

You're moving towards your wake

Enjoy Life

Before it's too, too late

notes

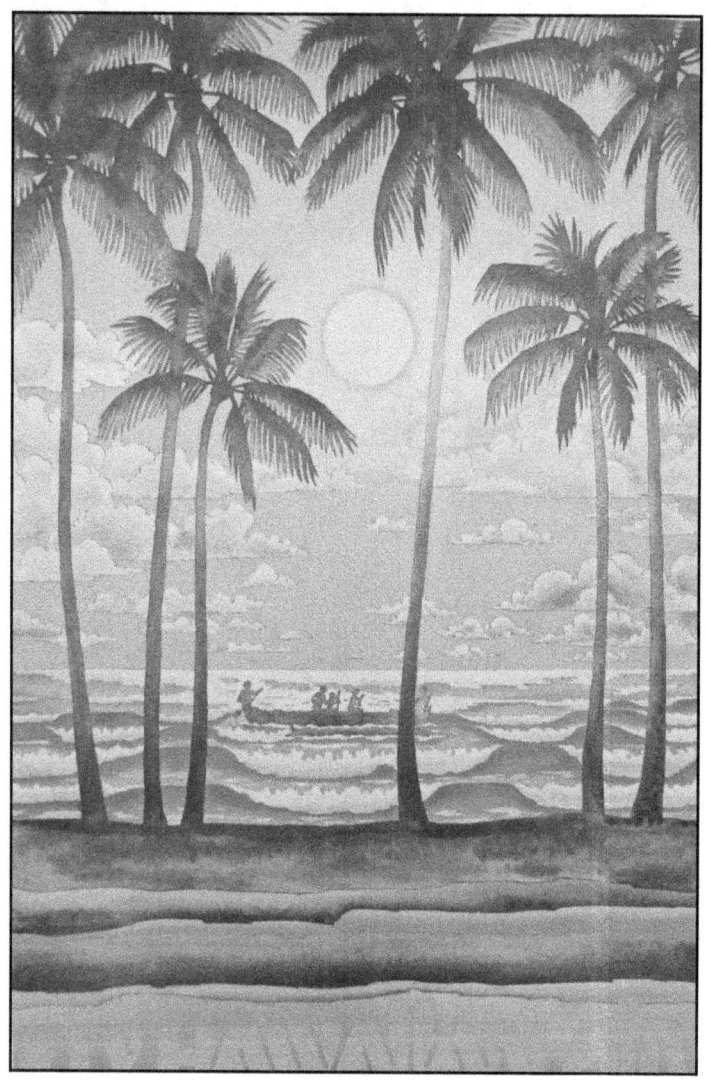

Visit us at:
www.deathhappenstoo.com